WHEN HEALTH IS LOST

Providing for the Costs of Long-term Nursing Home Care

WHEN HEALTH IS LOST

Providing for the Costs of Long-term Nursing Home Care

By

F. Bentley Mooney, Jr., Esquire

ISBN: 1-58721-531-4

This book is printed on acid free paper.

1stBooks – rev. 07/19/02

About the Book

In the mid-1980s, Congress became aware that many people -- almost one out of six -- work hard, live frugally, succeed in establishing a dignified standard of living as retirement age approaches, only to have that independence destroyed by the costs of long term care. To reach out to those left penniless by this *blitzkrieg*, Congress added several provisions -- optional to the states -- by which to become eligible for long term care under the Medicaid long term care program without first going broke. These provisions authorize certain transfers and do not count certain resources. They were added expressly to permit eligibility without spend-down, even permitting avoidance of lien recovery for benefits paid. All levels of government experienced continuing budgetary stress over the 15 year period ending in the late 1990s. During that time, characterization of these broken seniors shifted from "fine Americans, humbled by unfortunate circumstance" to "greedy geezers feeding at the public trough." *But Congress has seen fit to leave the eligibility planning rules in place.* We must therefore assume that the criticism is for public consumption while the *real* policy remains one designed to meet these important social needs.

Disclaimer

As we begin, a warning is necessary. This book conveys a principled approach to eligibility planning by which to shift the costs of long term nursing home care. Because your unique facts and circumstances weigh so heavily in making the legal decisions and personal choices involved, however, this book cannot be treated -- and is not intended -- as personal legal advice. Such advice may *only* be provided as part of a thorough legal examination of the facts, the law and objectives.

F. Bentley Mooney, Jr.

Acknowledgments

As you might imagine, writing a book while conducting a busy legal practice is an endeavor only for the industrious. The effort would have remained forever on the back burner but for the assistance of my long-time friend and secretary, Mee Y. Chang.

This book updates one I wrote in 1988. The reason for making the effort is at least in part attributable to those who see Medi-Cal eligibility planning as nothing more than enabling greedy geezers to feed at the public trough. When Americans who work hard for 50 years, pay their taxes and conduct their affairs with honor are broken by the costs of long term care for a loved one, that political rhetoric lends only outrage.

F. Bentley Mooney, Jr.

Table of Contents

Chapter Three

Chapter Four

Chapter Five

Accounting for the Special Needs Trust

Introduction

Herman pushed open the glass double doors of the doctor's office, stepped out into the fading colors of dusk, then hesitated by the steps leading to the parking lot. The voice was bouncing through his head like a bad commercial: "I'm sorry, Herman. She has Alzheimer's Disease. You can keep her at home for a few more months, but then she'll need long term care. You'd better budget four or five thousand dollars a month; those places don't come cheap."

His hand gripped the bannister with a slight tremor. "I just retired six months ago. One cruise, then this! We had so many plans. And how can I add four or five thousand dollars a month to our living expenses. We'll be broke in less than five years!"

Herman is not alone. You may face the same horrifying prospect; if not now, someday, and perhaps sooner than you think.

A study by the U.S. Department of Health and Human Services shows that people who reach age 65 face at least a 40% risk of entering a long term care facility. Although 45% of those nursing home stays last three months or less, more than one-third last a year or more; about 10% last five years or longer. In 1997, an estimated seven million people over the age of 65 needed long term care. By 2005, that number will increase to nine million, and by 2012, to 12 million.

Although the estimated national average cost for private patient care is on the order of $4,500 per month, in some parts of the country the costs can be twice that amount. Home care costs less, but is still costly. For an aide three times a week to help with dressing, bathing and preparing meals, the cost may be as much as $1,000 per month. Moreover, if skilled care is needed (like physical therapy), the costs are even greater.

Medicare pays for only 100 days of skilled and intermediate-level long term care, less than 2% of the total costs incurred. Private insurance pays a lesser percentage. The balance of the costs are paid from private savings and the various state-federal Medicaid programs.

Long term care insurance policies are actively marketed and serve this need well. More than 200 forms of coverage are now available. They remain, however, a minor factor compared to the total costs.

In California, Medi-Cal (this state's adaptation of the Medicaid program) is the *only* public health program that pays for long term care at the custodial level, or at the higher levels of care after the Medicare benefit expires.

Becoming eligible for Medi-Cal can require property transfers that are emotionally difficult for many. It can also lead to a sense of lost dignity. Consequently, Medi-Cal should be used only as a last resort. For many, however, it meets a critical need.

Often, Medi-Cal benefits can be combined with Supplemental Security Income (another state-federal program) to provide attractive benefits for a disabled person living in an assisted living facility (life care or room and board). For so long as assisted living meets the need, a long term care facility may be avoided.

In this book, you are provided with the background information needed in order to make an informed choice. Such critical decision-making must be based on sound information.

F. Bentley Mooney, Jr.

Chapter One

Disabled Adults:

A Social Problem Only Partly Addressed

Summary: *Lives are destroyed daily -- both economically and spiritually -- by stroke, Alzheimer's Disease, and other ailments requiring long-term care. Skilled and intermediate-level nursing home service is provided by Medicare for a limited period of time, but only Medicaid provides long-term and custodial care. A working knowledge of the major governmental health care programs is necessary to an understanding of Medi-Cal, the California Medicaid program. Advance planning may permit that applicant to both qualify and preserve lifetime economic security.*

For the most effective use of Medi-Cal, careful estate planning is essential. Chapter Three introduces this subject. Chapter Two explores alternatives to public social services, and this chapter provides context.

1.1 Governmental Health Care Programs

Medicare is a social insurance program for the elderly. It is not welfare, though some may argue the point in light of the way benefits and cost increases are allocated. Medicare is composed of two parts: Part A is hospital insurance and Part B is medical insurance. Even though Medicare coverage is fairly broad, 70% of its participants supplement it with "Medi-Gap" health insurance policies written by private companies.

Medicaid, which was established along with Medicare in 1965, is a welfare program of medical assistance to eligible needy persons. It is jointly funded and administered by the federal government and each of the states. The federal program serves as the guidelines to be followed in order for the states to obtain federal financial participation. Every state, plus Puerto Rico, Guam, the Virgin Islands and the Northern Mariana Islands, participates in Medicaid. Medicaid provides for long-term nursing care at all levels.

Medi-Cal is the California version of the Medicaid program. California treats everyone eligible for Supplemental Security Income as automatically eligible for Medi-Cal. For others, it provides generally liberal benefits, compared to many states.

For detailed information on Medicare, Medicaid and Medi-Cal, see *Appendix A*.

1.2 Historical Perspective

The Social Security Act was established in 1937 to provide old-age and survivors' income benefits. The benefits are payable to retired wage earners and their dependents or, if the wage earner is deceased, to that person's survivors. Later, disability income benefits were added and, in 1965, hospital and medical care under the Medicare program.

The Social Security Act was presented to the American people as an *insurance* program of benefits (though it was never required to establish and maintain legal reserves), not as a welfare program. This was an important political consideration in 1936, since most people at that time would move heaven and earth to avoid the indignity of accepting welfare. This must be much less so today, since the Congress now applies a "means test" by requiring those with incomes exceeding the federally-mandated threshold to report and pay income taxes on these formerly tax-free benefits.

As first conceived, the Social Security Act was intended to serve as a foundation in establishing financial independence. As such, it was never intended to fully satisfy retirement income needs or fully meet the support needs of dependents. Rather, the American people were cautioned to save, invest and purchase life and health insurance to supplement the benefits of Social Security. To a large extent, this view remains widely held.

To spread the cost of Social Security most fairly, the "taxable wage base" was established in the original act and remains today. The wage base has grown from $3,000 in 1937 to a figure approaching $100,000 today, and the *tax* on it has increased from 3% of earnings wage base in 1937 to 15.3% today (one-half paid by the employer). In addition, 1.45% of *all* earnings - not just the wage base - helps pay for medical costs under Medicare.

Medicare is aimed at acute care only. It was never intended to pay for comprehensive health care benefits, therefore it leaves almost wholly unaddressed the enormous costs of long term care.

The terms used to described levels of care in a nursing home are *skilled, intermediate* and *custodial.* They represent descending levels of medical services intensity. Skilled nursing facilities are those for which patients require registered nurses for at least two shifts daily for medication and emergency medical attention. Custodial nursing facilities are those for which patients do not require that level of attention from registered nurses, but *do* require assistance with dressing, bathing, eating, etc. Intermediate nursing facilities provide elements of both. Most convalescent hospitals and nursing homes have dropped their intermediate licenses, because reimbursement from Medicare and Medicaid is near those for custodial services; intermediate-level care cannot be provided at a profit in the absence of private resources to make up the difference.

Medicare pays less than 2% of nursing home care nationally, insurance even less. As a result, long-term care is paid mainly from personal savings, reducing thousands of Americans to abject poverty every year.

The cost of such care averages about $45,000 per year, and in most larger cities ranges up to more than $70,000. As far back as 1981, the cost of long term care nationally was $24 billion. The number of Americans over age 64, the primary users of these services, jumped from 29.9 million in 1983 to 35.3 million in 1990; 40.1 million were over 64 by 2000 and 66.3 million will be there in 2025. From 1985 to 1995, the *revenues* of long term care facilities grew at a rate of 3% per year, as the older population grew by 1½% per year in the same period.1 The *number* of such facilities, however, dropped by 23% This resulted in larger, consolidated long term care facilities, most operated by chain organizations. Since 1985, the length of long term care stays is down, and most facilities now serve niche markets; *e.g.*, post-hospital care, rehabilitation, ventilator care, etc. In short, long term care is moving in two directions: rehabilitation, and long term care of the profoundly disabled.

Of the roughly 40 million Americans over age 64 in 2000, nearly six million need -- or will need --long-term care, according to the National Center for Health Statistics.

Complicating all this is the situation facing the baby boomers, now often referred to as "the sandwich generation." These are the first to face the need to help parents for whom government programs may prove inadequate, and at the same time are required (or expected) to assist children through school and in getting started in life. With baby-boomer wives as well as husbands employed outside the home, few of them can stop work to care for an enfeebled parent.

More and more children today are forced by weak earnings and high housing costs to remain unmarried and live at home well beyond the school years. Many never become fully independent, some due to disabilities brought on by drug abuse, some due to developmental disabilities, some due merely to an apathetic attitude about career-building.

If Medicare does not pay for long term care, and if insurance is inadequate, unaffordable or unavailable, where do we turn to avoid the prospect of becoming both an economic and an emotional burden on our children as we grow older? We turn, from necessity, to Medicaid. While Medicare provides almost nothing, Medicaid can be all you need.

Medicaid is by far the largest third-party payor of long term care benefits. The federal government lays down the rules and provides partial funding, but to be available, the state in which the program participant resides must have adopted all or some part of the federal program.

The conventional wisdom holds that one must be impoverished to qualify for Medicaid, and technically that is true. The issue, however, is not as much the amount retained, but how it is held and who *gets* it. One view of life and success is to "learn the rules, then use them artfully." It is usually possible to transfer property in ways permitted by the Medicaid rules, qualify the applicant for long term care benefits (and perhaps SSI) and never permit the state to recover those health care costs from the transferred property.

Some view this approach as "morally offensive," One might suspect, however, that those holding such a view readily change them as soon as the problem becomes personal.

In the mid-1980s, Congress became aware that many people -- almost one out of six -- work hard, live frugally, succeed in establishing a dignified standard of living as retirement age approaches, only to have that independence destroyed by the costs of long term care. To reach out to those left penniless by this *blitzkrieg*, Congress added several provisions -- optional to the states -- by which to become eligible for long term care under Medicaid without total loss of economic security. These provisions authorize certain transfers and do not count certain resources. The new provisions were added expressly to permit eligibility without spend-down, even permitting avoidance of lien recovery for benefits paid. All levels of government experienced continuing budgetary stress over the 15-year period ending in the late 1990s. During that time, characterization of these broken seniors shifted from "fine Americans, humbled by unfortunate circumstance" to "greedy geezers feeding at the public trough." *But Congress saw fit to leave the eligibility planning rules in place.* We must therefore assume that the criticism is for public consumption while the *real* policy remains one designed to meet these important social needs.

In subsequent chapters, we will examine those rules. We will also examine private financing opportunities for those to whom such opportunities remain available.

1.3   Estate Planning Essentials

Any Medi-Cal planning must be accompanied by estate planning to some extent. Otherwise, the estate so saved may be lost, often by being left directly to the Medi-Cal participant (who is referred to throughout these pages as the "Applicant") or to the state. Following is a brief treatment of the usual estate planning issues and the various instruments used and useful in carrying out estate planning objectives. Complex estate planning rarely applies to the Applicant, but the methods constitute information you need as general background.

Wealth Transfer Taxes.   Congress enacted the first wealth transfer tax in 1913.   Its purpose was (and remains) to avoid concentrations of wealth among the fortunate few, with all the social stratification to which that leads.   The perfect picture is a society dominated by its middle class, people presumably happy in their circumstances, each with a pension, a tract home, two cars, an RV, a bass boat, four weeks' annual vacation and a good union.

People being people, however, many gave the economic well-being of their families a higher priority than the social goals of Congress.   The first taxpayer response was the regular transfer of wealth by means of lifetime gifts.   Congress then began taxing gifts in 1932.

Those taxpayers then began using trusts to bestow the economic benefits of capital on succeeding generations without subjecting that capital to taxation in the estates of those beneficiaries.   In response (with one false start), Congress enacted the generation-skipping transfer tax (GSTT) in 1986.

Those are about the only ways wealth transfers can be taxed. Today you and your spouse may make tax-free joint gifts to others of $20,000 per donee per year, and gifts to each other in unlimited amounts. The lifetime applicable exclusion amount for gift and estate tax is scaled to eventually reach $1 million in 2006. The exemption from GSTT is $1 million each for you and your spouse.

There are a number of ways the exclusions may be maximized, all with Congressional approval:

❑ **Gift Tax.** You may make annual gifts to children and others of $20,000 per year for each donee, effectively removing that capital from your gross estate (except for gift tax paid on gifts in excess of that amount and made in the final three years of life). You can also *leverage* those gifts which exceed $20,000 per donee in a number of ways. One is by giving the donee a remainder interest in a particular asset or fund, retaining a qualified right to its use or income for a term of years. In that transaction, the value of the gift is reduced by the present value of the retained interest, often producing a 60-80% discount on the gift tax involved. Another is by contributing annually to an irrevocable life insurance trust. $5,000 to $60,000 in premiums paid over some extended period of time buys perhaps $100,000 of cash to the children without income or estate tax.

❑ **Estate Tax.** You and your spouse may have community property (an undivided one-half interest in each asset). One or both of you may also have some separate property (premarital assets, gifts, inheritances). If you undertake *no* planning, all the community property and much of the separate property goes to the surviving spouse on the first death, usually with no estate tax. (The tax is excluded or is postponed by taking the unlimited marital deduction at the first death.) On death of the survivor, only the *survivor's* applicable exclusion amount is available.

However, with minimal planning, the applicable exclusion amount of the first spouse can be saved, effectively *doubling* the amount passing estate tax-free to or for the benefit of the family. This is accomplished by establishing a bypass trust at the first death. We trap a sum equal to the applicable exclusion amount in the bypass trust so it is not included in the gross estate of the survivor for estate tax purposes, then we use the marital deduction to postpone the estate tax on the remaining property interest of the deceased spouse. If you both survive to 2006, that maneuver alone enables you to avoid estate taxes on as much as $2 million. Of course, this is of no consequence to you, since the tax reduces the interest passing to the children; the effort is for *their* benefit. On the other hand, there are no great sacrifices involved, so it's nice of you to take care of them in this way.

The qualified terminable interest property trust (QTIP Trust) holds that portion of the deceased spouse's property interest that exceeds his or her applicable exclusion amount. With a death in 2001 and a $2 million community estate as an example, the survivor's community interest is allocated to the survivor's trust (revocable, amendable), $675,000 of the decedent's community interest is allocated to the bypass trust and the balance of the decedent's community interest -- $325,000 -- is allocated to the QTIP Trust. The preparer of the federal estate tax return (usually your trustee) is given an option whether or not to elect the estate tax marital deduction for the QTIP: if elected, tax is postponed and imposed at the survivor's death; if not, the tax is paid at the first death. Thus, if the surviving spouse has a long life expectancy, the marital deduction will ordinarily be taken, but if he or she has one foot in the grave and the other on a banana peel, it will not. Paying the tax separately at each death drives the tax into lower brackets for most estates. The QTIP Trust is, therefore, a post-death tax planning tool which also happens to semi-guarantee that the interest of the first spouse to die will be preserved for the children of that marriage and not blown by the next spouse.

❑ **Generation-Skipping Transfer Tax.** If you leave the estate to the children outright, or if you leave it in trust but give them the right to take it out, it will be included in their gross estates for federal estate tax purposes. But you can leave them the *income* from it and permit invasions of principal at the discretion of the trustee for needs that can be measured by an objective external standard (one sanctioned by the regulations is "reasonable care, support, health and education"). If you do, the trust estate will *not* be included and taxed in the estates of the children, grandchildren, and so on. By avoiding the estate tax every 20 years or so as another generation dies out and the benefits pass to the next one, major tax efficiency is introduced and capital may accumulated at a pace that stands a chance of beating the inflation rate. First-class educations, down payments on homes and other benefits may then be provided for up to five generations.

The fly in the ointment is GSTT. With planning, however, almost $3 million can be exempted from this tax, and the amount exempted is *never* burdened with a wealth transfer tax, no matter how much it appreciates in value. (That $3 million figure includes the use of a life insurance trust, where the leverage is enormous.)

The Plan. Here is how the plan operates:

❏ On death of the survivor (assuming the survivor has not left his or her portion of the estate to someone else or to the children in a different way), all three sub-trusts (bypass,

QTIP and survivor's) are consolidated for the benefit of the children, grandchildren and thereafter. If the combined $2 million GSTT exemption was effectively allocated, the portion of the remaining estate covered by it is held in the "GSTT Exempt Trust." If the estate is larger, that excess is allocated to a "GSTT *Non*exempt Trust." They have the same benefit structure.

❑ The exempt trust never pays a GSTT (assuming no drafting errors causing someone else to become a "deemed transferor," but I digress); it pays only *income* tax on retained trust earnings. This should permit it, with a solid total rate of return on investments, to both fund benefits for the beneficiaries and grow in value at a net after-tax rate exceeding the usual inflation rate.

❑ As to the *non*exempt trust, either the trust or the beneficiaries must pay a flat 55% GSTT on termination of a beneficiary's interest or on distribution. By separating the exempt from the nonexempt portions, we are able to charge *nontaxable* distributions (medical expenses and qualified tuition) and trust administration expenses to the nonexempt trust, and thereby

18

help the exempt trust to grow in value at a faster rate.

Keep in mind that the 1993 income tax changes compressed the tax brackets for the retained income of trusts. So long as those earnings are primarily from capital gains, however, the cost is manageable.

Trust Operation. Here are the management aspects of the various sub-trusts:

❏ The survivor's trust is revocable and may be amended so long as the survivor is alive and competent.

❏ The bypass and QTIP Trusts are irrevocable. The income of the QTIP Trust must be distributed only to the surviving spouse. The income from the bypass trust, however, may be accumulated and the trustee given power to invade for the benefit of the survivor, or it may be accumulated for later distribution to the children, or it may be distributed currently to either the children or the surviving spouse. The choices are usually driven by the income needs of the survivor: in large estates the bypass trust income is usually accumulated or distributed to the children; in medium-size estates it is more often distributed to the surviving spouse.

❑ Principal invasions are taken first from the survivor's trust (since that is the part not yet taxed), then from the QTIP Trust if the survivor's trust is exhausted, and from the bypass trust if both the survivor's and QTIP Trusts are exhausted.

❑ The spendthrift clause protects the surviving spouse from creditors to the extent of his or her beneficial interest in the QTIP and bypass trusts, and protects the children from creditors (and divorce) to the extent of their *entire* beneficial interests.

❑ With such a plan, and with professional management of the assets, a $1 million generation-skipping trust should throw off more than $24 million in benefits over five generations and grow to about $26 million in value. That is sufficient to keep it just ahead of a 2% average annual inflation rate. The *Rule Against Perpetuities* requires termination of the trust after about 90 years. Some states have repealed the rule, however, so it may be avoided by giving the trust a domicile on one of those states.

The Role of the Simple Will. Property of a decedent passes to the heirs in one of three ways:

❑ *By title* (typically joint tenancy right of survivorship).

❑ *By contract* (typically life insurance, pre-retirement pension benefits, IRAs, trusts).

❑ *By probate administration* (all the rest).

To the extent you fail to transfer assets to the trust, you risk the need for a probate administration proceeding with its attendant delays, expenses and loss of privacy.

One essential function of estate planning is to gather assets in one or two places for unified management. In most cases, those places are the family living trust and the irrevocable life insurance trust. Thus, the will serves as a fail-safe mechanism. If some assets are either overlooked or intentionally left outside the trust, the will picks them up and pours them over into the trust at the first death. It may be done by affidavit (no probate) if that portion of the estate is all *personal* property and worth less than $100,000 altogether. If the non-trust assets include an interest in real estate, or if it exceeds $100,000 in value, a probate proceeding is required in order to transfer it to the trust. So view the will as a *backup* tool, just in case a probate becomes necessary.

The Community Property Agreement. This instrument is intended to identify and validate the character of property as community and separate, to terminate unwanted joint tenancies, and to avoid adverse tax consequences in connection with irrevocable life insurance trusts.

As with the will, this serves in part as a fail-safe mechanism. By terminating unwanted joint tenancies, those former joint tenancy assets become probate assets. As such, the will can be used to transfer them to the trust after the first death.

The Irrevocable Life Insurance Trust. This kind of trust is a wonderful leverage device, but just as often comes under the heading of liquidity planning for the payment of estate taxes, or income replacement at premature death of the primary breadwinner.

The life insurance trust may be funded or unfunded. A funded trust is one to which you contribute income-producing property from which the life insurance premiums are paid. Because a contribution once made to the trust may not ordinarily be retrieved, funded life insurance trusts are rare.

An *un*funded irrevocable life insurance trust (ILIT) is one to which you and your spouse completely relinquish ownership and control of the policies, group life insurance certificates, or both. You do not retain a right to amend or revoke the trust and you cannot (without the right facts, a monumental effort and family-trustee cooperation) reclaim the policies and group certificates if you later change your mind.

Ordinarily, a family member should not serve as trustee; rather, you should name a corporate trustee. Those include bank trust departments and independent trust companies. A family member may serve well if both independent (*i.e.*, not a spouse or child living at home) and diligent enough to satisfy the withdrawal notice procedures discussed below. But if the trustee will be responsible for managing the proceeds for the benefit of your spouse, succeeding generations, or both, the legal and asset management obligations may prove overwhelming. That, in turn, may lead either to mismanagement or a last-minute substitution you would not appreciate if you were around to watch it happen.

A corporate trustee will charge an annual fee for holding the policies, receiving the premium notices, notifying you of the need for annual contributions, giving withdrawal notices to certain beneficiaries, then paying the premiums on lapse of the withdrawal rights. That fee is usually modest (considering the magnitude of the transaction) at around $600 to $900 per year.

As noted above, you would establish an ILIT for any of three reasons: cash to pay death taxes in order to avoid the forced sale of assets; income replacement if you die during your working years; and pure leveraged gifting.

There are three ways to pay estate taxes: from the estate (costs $1 for each dollar of tax); by borrowing (costs $1 *plus interest* for each dollar of tax); or with life insurance (costs 2¢ to 60¢ for each dollar of tax). Life insurance costs less and causes less disruption to the way the estate is held and operated; *e.g.*, it avoids the immediate need to dispose of closely-held business interests or real estate to raise funds for the tax man.

Unless the needs include income replacement, a survivor life insurance policy usually costs the least; it pays on death of the surviving spouse, making it available just nine months ahead of the tax bill.

If the trustee is *required* to pay your death taxes under the terms of the trust, that part of the life insurance proceeds so applied will be taxed as part of your estate. So instead the trustee is *authorized* to purchase assets from your estate at fair market value, or to loan money to the executor or trustee. The assets purchased or the notes received are then included in the ILIT estate, where they are held, managed and distributed for the named beneficiaries in accord with the trust terms.

As to income replacement, the single-life policy usually insures the primary breadwinner. At death of the insured, the trustee: (1) collects the proceeds, (2) invests them to generate income for the surviving spouse, and (3) if no surviving spouse, holds, manages and distributes in accord with the trust terms for children and beyond.

As to pure gift leverage, put the numbers to it. At age 60, for example, a single premium interest-sensitive life insurance policy will have a death benefit approximating 2.4 times the premium. If you set up six ILITs for six grandchildren, contribute $10,000 to each, with each trustee purchasing a $24,000 policy on your life, you have removed $60,000 from your gross estate for estate tax purposes and created $144,000 in additional capital for the benefit of those grandchildren. If the gifts are to charities, they may even be deductible. Assets tend to grow in value over time, so making a gift now will shift that appreciation to the donee, avoiding taxation in your estate.

When the trustee receives the policy or a cash contribution in trust, the interest of the trust beneficiaries is a "future interest." This is because they have no present rights at the time of the gift. As a future interest, the gift does not qualify for the $10,000 per donee annual gift tax exclusion.[2] It is important to obtain the annual exclusion because doing so reduces or eliminates the gift tax payable on transfer of the policy and on the contribution of annual premiums, also avoiding "unification" for estate tax purposes. The latter point is that by removing the premiums from your estate, it avoids pushing the estate remaining at your death into higher brackets.

To gain the annual exclusion, the trust agreement provides certain powers to withdraw all or part of the initial and annual trust contributions, based on *Crummey vs Commissioner*.[3] These powers are given in the trust agreement to certain people likely to receive benefits someday as remainder beneficiaries under the trust. In order, it comes up like this: the premium notice is received by the trustee as owner-beneficiary; the trustee notifies you that it is time to make your annual contribution; you do so; the trustee deposits the check in a trust bank account and sends a letter to the power holders (usually the children) notifying them that they may withdraw their proportionate interest if they do so within 30 days, and that otherwise the power will lapse; the power holders (being intelligent and understanding people) decline to take the cash, after which the trustee pays the premium with it. The existence of the power to withdraw makes the gift one of a "present interest," giving rise to the annual gift tax exclusion for trust contributions.

As a general rule, a policy insuring your life is owned by and payable to the trustee of your ILIT and will not be included in your gross estate for federal estate tax purposes. However, the proceeds *will* be included if you retain any incidents of ownership in the policy at the time of death, whether exercisable by you alone or in conjunction with another person or entity.[4] Such incidents include the right to borrow the cash values, change settlement options, change the beneficiary, surrender the policy, change dividend options and assign the policy as collateral.

The present IRS position on assigned *group* life insurance is that the death proceeds are not included in your estate *if*: you make a lifetime assignment, including all your incidents of ownership; both the group master policy and state law permit such an absolute assignment of ownership, including the assignment of any conversion rights; and the policy cost is funded entirely by the employer.5

One final caveat: when you transfer ownership of *existing* life insurance into the ILIT, you must live three years beyond the date of assignment in order to avoid inclusion of those proceeds from your gross estate for federal estate tax purposes.6 On the other hand, if the trustee purchases *new* insurance on your life, exclusion is immediate.

Any gift tax paid on policy assignments and ILIT contributions made within three years of death are included in your gross estate.7 This militates in favor of using permanent forms of life insurance and working to get them fully paid up at some point early in the game. As to federal *income* tax considerations, the trustee takes your status with respect to the policy. Thus, if the proceeds are income tax free to you, they are income tax free to the trustee.

The ILIT is an important tool in estate planning. If the net estate plus life insurance exceeds the applicable exclusion amount, the first defensive move is to employ the marital deduction trust discussed earlier, effectively doubling the amount excluded from taxation. If the net estate plus life insurance exceeds the *combined* applicable exclusion amounts, the next logical step is to remove the life insurance from your gross estate, thereby effectively saving taxes at the margin (up to 55%). By that means, the ILIT can mean major tax savings.

Durable Power of Attorney. The durable power of attorney is a creature of statute that sanctions a twist on the generic form. Let's track it through to this modern application.

A generic power of attorney is a written instrument given by a *principal* to an *agent* (the latter historically called the "attorney-in-fact") authorizing the agent to perform certain specified acts on behalf of the principal. It may be as detailed as collecting income, maintaining books of account, managing property, paying bills, reporting taxes and accounting periodically to the principal, or it may be as simple as authorizing grandparents to obtain emergency medical care for a grandchild they are taking on a vacation trip.

The power of attorney may have a specified term, or may provide that it continues until revoked. It terminates upon the expiration of any specified term, or by operation of law on the death or incompetence of the principal, whichever first occurs.

All or most states have enacted statutes authorizing and recognizing *durable* powers of attorney. These are powers of attorney that continue in effect if the principal becomes incompetent. To be "durable," a specific provision is required. Here is a typical provision:

> "By this document I intend to create a durable power of attorney for health care as authorized by the *California Probate Code*. This power of attorney shall remain in force despite my subsequent incapacity."

A variation on the durable power of attorney is now in common use: the *springing* durable power of attorney. Here, the terms of the authority granted are set when signed, but the authority of the agent is delayed until the day arrives when the principal is no longer competent or otherwise able to express an opinion on the subject matter. In effect, the principal has granted *no* authority while able to act on the subject matter personally, and the agent merely stands in the wings, ready to take over if, as, or when required. This is the usual form for a durable power of attorney for *health care*, and frequently employed for durable powers of attorney for *property*.

In the durable power of attorney for health care, you: (1) name the agent authorized to act on your behalf in dealing with health care providers, along with one or more alternate agents; (2) define "health care decision"; (3) express your wishes in connection with life support systems, nutrition and hydration; (4) name a person (usually the agent) to serve as conservator of your person if one is ever needed; and (5) both authorize and express your wishes with respect to releasing medical records, signing waivers and releases, autopsy, gift of body parts and burial arrangements.

Some people use a *Directive to Physician* on the matter of life support systems. Although it may be coordinated with the power of attorney, it adds little.

Conclusion. Often coming into play are lifetime gifts, business buy-sell agreements, charitable gifts, inter-generational sales, private annuities and valuation discount arrangements. Plan specifics are driven by your personal facts and circumstances. This, however, should serve to orient you to the tools most often employed in estate planning.

Chapter Two

Private Funding

for Long-Term Nursing Care

Summary: *In "Endless Care with Costs to Match," (Insight, Dec. 28, 1987-Jan. 4, 1988, p.44), Richard P. Teske, Deputy Assistant Secretary for Public Affairs at the federal Department of Health and Human Services (DHHS) is quoted as calling proposed publicly-funded long-term nursing home care, "... an entitlement program for middle and upper-income people." Mr. Teske also pointed out that, "Entitlement programs already in place threaten to bankrupt the U. S. Treasury over the long run." If these statements fairly depict the attitude of DHHS (and little has changed except for election-year rhetoric), it is clear that no new help is in prospect from the federal government.*

To the extent public programs do not fund the cost of long term care, that burden falls on the private sector -- your savings and your insurance. It is your economic security that we wish to preserve, so let us here examine the market for long term care insurance and a few other tools for meeting that need.

2.1 Long-Term Care Insurance

Private nursing care insurance was first made available in the late 1970s. The insurance companies' early experience taught them that underwriting this business requires caution in every respect.[8] Most applicants were found to be over 70 years of age and already showing signs of debilitating disease. Because insurance companies cannot operate profitably by insuring people clearly about to become claimants, premiums quickly jumped to unaffordable levels. Those premium levels were held in check only by not covering pre-existing conditions. Private insurance remains, however, one of the most promising vehicles for spreading the costs of long-term nursing care widely enough to economically meet the requirements of those in need.

One obvious fact cannot be ignored: in order for long term care policies to be affordable and to also provide full coverage, more Americans must purchase them earlier in life. Only by that means will the risks be spread widely enough through the over-64 population to bring about the required economies of scale. As this book is written, only 2% of this group maintains long-term care insurance.

In one study[9], it was estimated that Medicaid expenditures would be reduced by 23% if only one-half of those between ages 65 and 69 would purchase long-term care insurance. According to the Health Insurance Association of America,[10] such insurance is affordable *right now* to middle class Americans over age 64; these are the very ones who would be financially destroyed by the costs of long term care. The association estimates that 80% of those between age 65 and 69 can purchase such insurance at a premium less than 10% of income, and 50% of them could do it with less than 5% of income.

The insurance industry began in the mid-80s to recognize long term care insurance as a $50 billion market. As a result more than 80 commercial carriers and 12 Blue Cross/Blue Shield plans were in the long-term care market by the end of 1988, up from 16 in 1983. This competition is the market force that stabilized rates at generally affordable levels and brought about significant improvement in the quality of coverage. Today, more than 100 carriers are marketing long term care policies.

For a list of insurance companies selling long-term care insurance in California, contact the Health Insurance Association of America, 1001 Pennsylvania Avenue N.W., Washington, DC 20004.

Before you purchase a policy, check the rating of the insurance company with A.M. Best Company's rating service. It provides an objective opinion of financial stability and management quality. Less than one-half of the companies in this market carry a high Best's rating. That does not mean you assume an unjustified risk in purchasing their policies, but it is a consideration.

The State of California has also introduced its *California Partnership for Long Term Care*. It established feature and quality standards, along with fair pricing levels, for insurance covering long term care in custodial facilities, adult day care, home, board and care, assisted living facilities. The incentive offered to consumers is a liberalized Medi-Cal Property Reserve, generally increasing the value of assets the Applicant may retain while obtaining Medi-Cal eligibility for long term care by a sum equal to the aggregate insurance benefits. So far, only a handful of carriers have obtained state approval for their plans; all are financially sound organizations. State certification assures the buyer that the plan contains all the features and makes available all the services marked with an "*" at a fair and reasonable cost.

For materials on the program, write to:

The California Partnership for Long Term Care
714 P Street, Room 616
Sacramento, California 95814

or call (800) CARE 445. Its website is http://www.dhs.ca.gov/cpltc.

All long-term nursing care policies now on the market are written on a daily indemnity form, much like the more familiar hospital indemnity plan. Daily benefits range up to $120 or more during confinement, and are paid for periods ranging in length from one to four years or more. To put this in context, 95% of all nursing home stays are terminated by discharge or death within four years.

In order to gain a sense for the rate of increase in long term care costs, here are the averages for California over the last couple of decades:

Year	One Day	One Year
1980	$ 42	$15,330
1990	88	32,120
1998	130	47,450

The premium level is a function of several facts:

1.2 Age is the most important factor. The rates increase with age.

❑ The elimination period (deductible) reduces the premium if longer and increases it if shorter.

❑ The daily benefit level reduces the premium if lower and increases it if higher.

❑ The pay period increases the premium if longer and reduces it if shorter.

❑ Additional features increase the premium.

❑ Spousal discounts are often available when both spouse purchase policies through the same company.

❑ Group discounts may be available when the policy is purchased through an employer-sponsored or association group plan.

Each company set its own rates, but here are some examples that serve to give you a general idea as to the costs involved:

Amount of Coverage	Premium, Purchase at 50	Premium, Purchase at 65
$ 80,000	$470 or more	$1,070 or more
120,000	560 or more	1,310 or more
200,000	740 or more	1,730 or more

In 1987, The Brookings Institute calculated the national average annual cost for out-of-home nursing care at $22,000. That cost reflected a 20-year price escalation at the rate of 15% per year. By extending increases at that rate, the institute estimated that by 2017, those annual costs will be $119,000. The point to be taken is that the daily indemnity levels under the policies now on the market are often fixed; *i.e.*, they do not increase to match rising nursing home costs. If possible, then, you should purchase policies containing an inflation-adjustment feature so the benefit payments keep pace with rising costs.

In order to avoid insuring sick people who immediately submit claims, the insurance companies (and Blue Cross/Blue Shield, for that matter) employ medical underwriting in ways ranging from tight to liberal. Waivers of coverage for pre-existing health conditions are widely and routinely used. At the time a claim is submitted, the company may look back as far as five years to identify health conditions that were not disclosed at the time of the application. It may then characterize some of them as pre-existing conditions permitting denial of the claim. *Full* policy coverage (that is, where the company cannot look back) may be provided from six months to two years after the policy is issued.

Most health insurance policies contain standard exclusions for acts of war, suicide and attempted suicide. The major difference between health insurance generally and long-term nursing care policies in particular is the coverage of mental illness. Older policy forms exclude it, even those mental illnesses which are organic in nature (*e.g.*, senility and Alzheimer's Disease). Most modern forms of coverage, however, cover mental illness fully.

Careful attention must be given to admissions requirements. Many older-form policies require a three-day stay in an acute care facility for the same or related condition before paying for convalescent care in a nursing home. The intent is to assure the insurance company of the medical necessity. Others gain that assurance by requiring the insured to pay a deductible measured in terms of days, not dollars. Such companies will start payments in 20 to 100 days after admission, with options for longer periods so as to enable the insured to plan around the 100 days of skilled nursing level of care generally available from Medicare.

One more suggestion: insist on a policy that is guaranteed renewable. Renewability features fall generally into three categories:

❑ **Commercial:** The insurance company can cancel your policy whenever it pleases (*e.g.*, right after the first claim).

❑ **Guaranteed Renewable:** The insurance company cannot cancel the policy or refuse to renew it as long as you pay your premiums on time. Moreover, it cannot raise your premium rate unless it raises the rates at the same time for every insured with the same policy.

❑ **Noncancellable and Guaranteed Renewable**: The same as guaranteed renewable, except that the insurance company may not raise your premium on *any* basis. To date, no such policy provision is available in the nursing home care market, but competitive pressures may one day bring it to pass.

2.2 Life Insurance Arrangements for Nursing Home Care

Given a promising new market, insurance industry ingenuity knows few limits. For example, First Penn-Pacific Life Insurance Company (2021 Midwest Road, Oak Brook, Illinois 60521, (312) 495-3336) and others are approved in California to sell a life insurance policy that pays nursing home expenses from *death* benefits. Under most life insurance policy forms, only the cash *surrender* value is available for long-term care expenses. There is no requirement that you die first, or that you first be admitted to an acute care facility in order to start the nursing home benefits. 100% of the face amount is available and there is no waiting period before benefits begin.

The features vary widely from carrier to carrier. Ask your agent to present a representative sample of the available plans.

2.3 Cash Accumulation Plans

Cash accumulation plans range from the reserving a specific fund of cash for long term care, to special purpose plans. Among the former: Individual Retirement Accounts, annuities and home equity conversions. Among the latter: Individual Medical Accounts and VEBAs -- Voluntary Employee Beneficiary Associations. Following is a brief description of each:

Individual Retirement Accounts (IRA). These are creatures of federal tax law, used for tax-favored accumulation of cash during the working years. They are structured as trust or custodial accounts for the exclusive benefit of the account holder and beneficiaries.[11] IRAs may be established by contributions or by rollover of sums received from qualified plans or from other IRAs. Non-rollover contributions are limited to $2,000 per year and are deductible for income tax purposes if the account holder is not a participant in a qualified retirement plan at the time of the contribution. If the account holder's income is low enough, he or she may deduct the contribution even if participating in a qualified plan. Income of the IRA accumulates tax-deferred, and the tax is imposed on distribution. A penalty generally applies to distributions made prior to attainment of age

59½. Distributions must be taken starting in the year after attaining age 70½

Roth Individual Retirement Accounts (Roth IRA). This is another form of IRA.[12] Annual contributions are also limited to $2,000 ($4,000 for married taxpayers filing jointly), reduced by any amount contributed to a regular IRA. The maximum contribution is phased out for married taxpayers filing jointly with income from $150,000-160,000, single taxpayers with incomes from $95,000-110,000, and married taxpayers filing separately with incomes from $0-10,000. Rollover contributions are permitted, but not for taxpayers with incomes over $100,000 (single or married, and regardless of reporting status). Annual contributions are not deductible.[13] Furthermore, rollover contributions are generally taxed to the account holder in the year of the rollover.[14] The offsetting advantage of the Roth IRA is that, unlike a regular IRA, qualified distributions are completely excluded from taxable income of the account holder or other beneficiary.[15] Generally, fewer restrictions apply. For example: the maximum contribution is not affected by the availability of qualified retirement plans; contributions may be made after age 70½; and there are no required distributions.16

Because these accounts are segregated from all other funds, it is conceptually easy to reserve them for the infirmities of old age, including long term care costs.

Annuities and Life Insurance Without the Long Term Care Feature. Annuities and traditional forms of life insurance fall into the same category. The problem is that the savings accumulated are generally too small to be useful. A survey conducted in 1984 jointly by the American Council of Life Insurance and the Life Insurance Marketing and Research Association disclosed that the median amount of life insurance (death benefit, not cash value) was only $13,000 for men and $5,000 for women. Cash surrender values are generally less than one-half the death benefit, sums that hardly begin to fund long-term care costs.

Home Equity Conversions. These are financing transactions intended to liquidate the homeowner's equity while permitting the homeowner to continue living in the home. The most discussed transactions are reverse mortgage and sale-leaseback arrangements. In the reverse mortgage, the lender pays monthly installments to the owner-borrower, and the installments are secured by a deed of trust on the home. The total of the installments to be paid is limited to the usual percentage of value in more typical real estate loans, and must be repaid or renegotiated when the owner lives out her life expectancy or on sale of the property, whichever first occurs.

In the sale-leaseback, the owner sells the property to an investor and leases it back for a term usually measured by the owner-seller's life expectancy. The lease payments and carrying costs can affect the price, depending on whether it is higher or lower than market rates.

A similar transaction is one in which (1) the fair market value of the property is ascertained, (2) IRS tables establishing life estate and remainder interests at various ages are consulted, (3) carrying costs over the owner-seller's life expectancy are estimated, using insurance industry annuity tables to determine life expectancy, (4) the owner sells the property to an investor, reserving a life estate (the right to occupy and to receive all rents, issues and profits from it during the seller's lifetime) for a price discounted from the remainder interest to account for the obligation assumed by the investor to pay all insurance, taxes and maintenance costs. For example: Assume the house is worth $100,000, the life estate is $15,000, and the carrying costs are estimated at $3,000 per year for a 10-year life expectancy. The investor might pay $55,000 cash plus $3,000 per year (estimated) for as long as the owner-seller lives, expecting that the owner-seller will die in 10 years, terminating the reserved life estate and leaving the investor with the property, free and clear.

While home equity conversions offer large numbers of older Americans an attractive method of financing their long term care needs, most are hesitant to encumber their homes. Moreover, due to the limited number of conversions to date, we lack enough information to fully evaluate its potential for this purpose.

The Medical Savings Account. This vehicle is aimed precisely at funding medical expenses. Contributions are deductible in a manner similar to IRAs. Interest earnings are tax-deferred until the account holder attains the age of 65. There is no penalty on withdrawal so long as the distribution is to pay for some health care expense of the account holder or family member. There is no contribution offset for participation in IRAs or other qualified plans. The maximum contributions are $1,462 for an individual and $3,375 for a family.

VEBAs. These are *employer*-sponsored accumulation vehicles, thus probably unavailable to you. So, we will leave them undiscussed.

2.4 Other Long-Term Care Financing Vehicles

Among the remaining means of financing long-term nursing care costs, two stand out: social/health maintenance organizations (S/HMOs) and life care communities.

These organizations provide *services*, rather than *indemnity* payments to other health care providers. This is the characteristic distinguishing them from insurance forms of financing. Since they provide both the costs and the services, it is in their interests to operate economically. That built-in incentive leads to preventive techniques and low-cost choices among available options in providing needed care most economically.

S/HMOs. These organizations provide a package of medical and long term care services, enlarging (to the extent of long-term care) the benefits available under Medicare. The members pay a monthly fee, most of which is reimbursed by Medicare. While enrolled in the S/HMO, members must receive all their hospital and medical services through that provider.

As a relatively new development on the social needs financing scene, S/HMOs are still in the test stage. When the original version of this book was written (in 1988), they were operating as demonstration projects at Long Beach, California, Portland, Oregon, Minneapolis, Minnesota and Brooklyn, New York. Each site served about 4,000 enrollees. All are struggling. The Long Beach S/HMO, established in 1984, is called the *SCAN Health*

Plan. It attempted in April 1997 to go private as a means of securing fresh capital so as to remain independent. Part of the problem is due to federal limits on expansion, part to the competitiveness of the managed health care industry, but some must also be attributable to the difficulty of managing the expense of long term care. To switch to for-profit status, Long Beach must fund a charitable foundation with the distribution of excess assets. State regulators questioned its proposal in that regard, stalling its attempts to compete by restructuring itself.

Supporters of the S/HMO approach contend that they can allocate needed health care services to their members humanely and efficiently, that they can prevent overutilization by serving as both provider and gatekeeper, and that their case management approach permits better management of the acute and long-term care services. Proponents also point out that S/HMOs deliver services to their members without requiring relocation to a more expensive skilled nursing facility or retirement home, and without requiring sale of the family home or other lifestyle disruptions.

One might wonder about the obvious temptation to skew choices toward those services reimbursed by Medicare, including perhaps artful rationalizations of the need for Medicare-financed skilled care nursing facilities, and away from the long-term and custodial services paid from that portion of the monthly fee allocated to extended care (the part the S/HMO gets to keep if not spent). Such a pattern, widely existing, could have a profoundly deleterious effect on the public costs of health care. Only time will tell.

Life Care Communities. These organizations are also known as "continuing care communities." They provide not only the hospital, medical and long-term care obtainable from S/HMOs, but housing as well. This package of services is provided in exchange for an entrance fee (generally ranging from $7,500 to $100,000) and monthly service fees (generally ranging from $1,000 to $3,000).

Most life care communities are organized in housing complexes of 200 to 250 units, and include in the package emergency medical care, long term care, meals, recreational programs, transportation and other services. New members are generally able to walk and care for themselves in their own apartment or townhouse. As physical condition begins to deteriorate, they are moved to assisted living or long term care sections for higher levels of care.

The entrance fee was largely non-refundable in the early years. Modernly, however, it is refunded *pro rata* for death or departure during the first five years.

If you consider a life care community, investigate its financial condition and the availability of a partial refund of the entrance fee upon death or departure. You should also balance the financial condition of the life care community against the extent to which it guarantees not to increase monthly service fees. Specifically, a life care community that guarantees its rates years into the future without reserving a way to cover increasing costs, may be headed for trouble, taking your money with it. One with a sound balance sheet, operating at a profit, and which reserves the right to increase monthly fees, however, may be a good long-term prospect; especially if it will refund a large part of your entrance fee in the event increased monthly fees turn out to be unaffordable.

Life care communities offer quite a few advantages: a positive social environment, organized activities and lifetime residential and health care. Because only people in good health view life care communities as a sound financial move (believing they will live long enough to beat the system), life care community residents are generally in better health and live longer than their non-life care community-resident peers.

S/HMOs, life care communities and other service programs not yet conceived, offer important potential for effectively meeting public needs for long term care. Their case management approach is now a proven method for providing extended care humanely and economically, in a risk-sharing, prepaid mode of operation. Further refinement and growth of S/HMOs and life care communities should be encouraged.

Chapter Three

Planning Specifics

Summary: *Be careful about conflicts of interest in the planning process. Life is often better if you can avoid Medi-Cal altogether; but for those who require it, there is usually a way. The basic planning technique is to transfer assets into exempt categories so they can be given away without penalty, and otherwise transfer and plan around a period of ineligibility.*

The preceding chapters provide the background information and context for the specific planning techniques described here. Our purpose is to use every practical and legal means to protect your assets and those of your loved ones from the economic *blitzkrieg* of long-term care.

3.1 Introduction

To be useful, this book cannot serve as an exhaustive treatise on every conceivable planning rule and maneuver. Rather, we address those applicable to common fact situations.

This area of the law changes frequently, so all such planning should be undertaken only with thoughtful guidance from an advisor familiar with the Medi-Cal long term care program and related public benefits law. Unfortunately, various non-lawyer marketing groups have surfaced in recent years, the purpose of which is to sell trusts and annuities by means of incorrect, incomplete and misleading representations. Protect yourself by dealing only with a qualified elder law attorney.

3.2 Conflicts of Interest.

The primary purpose of Medi-Cal eligibility planning is to preserve the lifetime economic security of the Applicant. That process involves the transfer of assets in ways that incidently save the inheritance of the children.

The planning may therefore be misunderstood as an inheritance preservation procedure, rather than for its true aim. This also introduces the possibility of a conflict of interest. Suppose the children engage the attorney to advise on implications of the approaching incapacity of a parent. The process may involve gifts to the children, and the children may wish to create a special needs trust for the Applicant- parent and fund it with the assets received by gift. In that case, the attorney must decide who is to be the client: the Applicant-parent or the children. This is because the property transfers may be made for reasons that differ, or even change in mid-transaction. The attorney cannot represent both the Applicant and the children-donees without full disclosure and a written informed waiver of the potential adverse interests, due to the conflicting fiduciary duties owed to each. Therefore, good practice would be for the Applicant to be the client in virtually all cases in which he or she is competent. If that party is *not* competent, a court proceeding will be required in order to lawfully make the property transfers, and the court will appoint independent counsel to advise and protect the rights of the Applicant.

Where representing the spouse or children of an incompetent Applicant, the attorney must provide to any who are *former* clients an opportunity to obtain independent counsel, so as to be able to protect their interests in the planning choices to be made. Otherwise, those former clients must either proceed without representation or consent in writing to the joint representation of adverse interests.

3.3 Avoid Medi-Cal if Possible

Most of us spend our working lives preparing to retire at a dignified standard of living. Where possible, planning for long term care should be conducted with that same goal in mind. That goal may not matter much if finances dictate the choices, or if the mental condition of the Applicant is such that *no* luxury can be appreciated; but where there *is* a choice, consider avoiding Medi-Cal altogether: the planning requires asset transfers that can be disturbing.; and the anxiety is compounded by moving from familiar surroundings. Consequently, you should reflect at length on whether home care, the use of a life care community or a Social/Health Maintenance Organization (S/HMO) is feasible.

The life care community may be feasible if, for example, the Applicant owns a home and little else. If a home loan, sale or remainder interest sale will produce enough cash for the entrance fee, and if the home may be rented for an amount sufficient to cover debt service and other home-related expenses, and if other income (Social Security retirement benefits, pension income, interest, cash flow from the house rental, etc.) is sufficient to fund the monthly charges, the life care community may be the perfect choice.

If the Applicant placed in an life care community or S/HMO program is legally competent, routine estate planning should be undertaken. That will ordinarily include a living trust to gain skilled management of property interests and a durable power of attorney to obtain sympathetic representation in making vital residential and health care choices.

If the Applicant placed in an life care community or S/HMO is unmarried and *not* legally competent, a probate conservatorship proceeding should be commenced. The conservator is vested with substantially the same legal powers as the trustee and the attorney-in-fact noted in Chapter One. The major differences are that the conservator must obtain court approval of the estate management each year and the conservatorship estate must be distributed in a probate administration proceeding at the death of the applicant as conservatee. With court approval, though, estate planning may also be undertaken in order to establish a trust by which to avoid probate administration.

3.4 Eligibility Requirements for the Medi-Cal Long Term Care Program

First, we must separate this discussion from some related areas. Medi-Cal automatically pays for hospital-medical services for those who qualify for Supplemental Security Income. It also provides medical coverage to those who otherwise qualify for a cash grant welfare program. Furthermore, Medi-Cal also provides in-home support services. Each of these areas come with eligibility rules different from those for long term care.17 We here deal with none of those fact situations. Rather, this discussion is limited to the long term care program.

After considering all the private options, long term care under the Medi-Cal program may be the logical choice. If so, you must address the basic aim of planning for Medi-Cal eligibility: *to get it without first going broke.*

The Applicant is entitled to Medi-Cal (including the full cost of long term care) when (1) *nonexempt assets* are within the allowed value (Property Reserve), *and* (2) when institutionalized. You need *both*, although the planning often precedes institutionalization by months or years, with application following.

The Property Reserve is $2,000 for the Applicant and $4,000 combined when both applicant and spouse are applying for long term care coverage. If the Applicant is married, the non-disabled spouse is entitled to retain a much larger amount as the Community Spouse Resource Allowance. He or she may own up to $60,000 in non-exempt assets (adjusted annually for inflation) without loss of eligibility for the Applicant.[18] Community and separate property distinctions are ignored in determining the amount of the Community Spouse Resource Allowance, so it matters not that the Applicant spouse has no ownership of the Community Spouse's separate property.[19] The determination is based on the assets held by the Applicant and Community Spouse in the month in which the application is received by the county (Snapshot Rule).[20] The importance of this rule is that the Community Spouse may receive and own assets in any amount, as long as they are acquired after the month in which the application is submitted.

3.5 Important Terms.

In order to better understand the planning concepts discussed in the remainder of this chapter, the following key terms must be explained:

❑ **Community Spouse/Individual's Spouse.** Both terms refer to the spouse who is not disabled. *Prior* to institutionalization of the Applicant, he or she is called the "Individual's Spouse." *After* institutionalization, the

Individual's Spouse becomes the "Community Spouse." See pages 66-67 for the purpose in drawing this distinction.

❑ **Community Spouse Resource Allowance.** The amount of counted assets the Community Spouse is allowed to own without loss of eligibility for the Applicant spouse.

❑ **"Eligible for a Day, Eligible for the Whole Month."** A California Department of Health Services (DHS) rule under which any fraction is dropped in calculating a period of Medi-Cal eligibility.[21]

❑ **Minimum Monthly Maintenance Needs Allowance.** An amount, originally set at $1,500 per month and adjusted for inflation, which represents the minimum needed by the Community Spouse for a dignified standard of living. It is used in determining how much of the Applicant's income must be allocated to the Community Spouse in order to bring that spouse to this level (or as close to it as a 100% allocation will permit).

❑ **"Name on the Check Rule."** Under the *Medicare Catastrophic Care Act of 1988*

(MCCA), income is attributable to the spouse whose name appears on the check or other instrument representing that income. If both spouse's names are on the instrument, the income item is divided between them. Income payments from a trust are considered income to the spouse to whom the payments are actually made. These income rules apply regardless of any state laws relating to community property.[22]

❑ **Personal Needs Allowance.** For Medi-Cal beneficiaries in long term care, this allowance of $35 per month is taken from income otherwise applied to Share of Cost (see below). It is intended to meet needs that are not funded by the long term care program; *e.g.*, hair care, reading materials, television, day trips, etc.[23]

❑ **Share of Cost.** Although there is no income limit with respect to Medi-Cal eligibility, a long term care program participant cannot receive Medi-Cal benefits unless almost all monthly income is spent on medical expenses. The part of the income that must be spent on medical care before Medi-Cal will pay is called "share of cost."

After redeploying assets as part of the eligibility planning engagement, most passive income is received with the name of the Community Spouse or the trustees of a Special Needs Trust on the check. Therefore, only Social Security, Railroad Retirement and pension income remains (in most cases) with the Applicant's name on the check. From that amount, the Personal Needs Allowance and personal medical insurance premiums are deducted, then part may be allocated to the Community Spouse (if there *is* a Community Spouse and if his or her income is less than the Minimum Monthly Maintenance Needs Allowance); the rest is the Applicant's Share of Cost.

3.6 Asset Classification

The asset categories are "counted resources," "exempt assets" and assets "deemed unavailable."

Exempt Assets. Those assets which are *excluded* from the Property Reserve -- thus not counted in determining eligibility -- are described in *California Code of Regulations* as "exempt assets." Those treated as exempt in determining eligibility for Medi-Cal, *without limit as to value*, include the following:

❑ The residence of the Applicant, if an intent to return is stated in the Medi-Cal application at Question 17A and no order to the contrary is made after a fair hearing;[24]

❑ The sale proceeds of the residence, for a period of six months after the closing;[25]

❑ Heirloom jewelry;[26]

❑ One motor vehicle, if used primarily to transport the Applicant;[27]

❑ Furniture, fixtures, appliances and other household effects located at the residence of the Applicant;[28]

❑ Personal effects of the Applicant;[29]

❑ Recreational equipment (golf clubs, etc.);[30]

❑ Musical instruments;[31]

❑ Burial insurance;[32]

❑ Burial trust or prepaid burial contract;[33]

❑ Burial plots, vaults and crypts, if purchased by the Applicant for personal use or for "any member of the family" (an undefined term);[34] and

❑ *Perhaps* real property used wholly or partly for self-support.[35]

❑ The assets of a business (equipment, inventory, licenses and materials) are exempt as long as the business is earning a profit of 6% or more on net assets. Working capital is also exempt for an amount up to three times average monthly expenses.[36] To utilize this exemption, get a statement from your accounting professional along the following lines:

TO WHOM IT MAY CONCERN:

With respect to the cash requirements of [Client name]'s business, [Name of business], the monthly operating cash requirements average

approximately $ [   ].   This is
based on operations for the period
[Date] to [Date].

Operating expenses consist of
[List]. Being a seasonal business,
the expenses range from $[ ] to $[
].

If further information is required,
contact me at [ ].

Sincerely,

[Name of Accountant]

Other categories of assets having *limited value
exempt status* include life insurance, if the
aggregate face value (not surrender value) does
not exceed $1,500.[37] If it exceeds that figure,
the cash surrender value is counted in
determining eligibility.

Assets Deemed "Unavailable."   Assets
"deemed unavailable" to the Applicant for
Medi-Cal eligibility purposes, thus not
considered, are those which cannot be reduced
to cash within a reasonable period of time and

those over which the Applicant has no control. Neither the statutes nor the cases define "availability." We must therefore turn to federal law as incorporated in our *California Welfare and Institutions Code*.38 At the federal level, it is addressed in the *Omnibus Budget Reconciliation Act of 1987*39 (OBRA '87), amending Section 1613(b) of the *Social Security Act*.40 Deemed unavailable assets include *at least* the following:

❑ The (otherwise) countable resources of a *Special Needs Trust*, if the trust was *not* established *by* the Applicant or by the *spouse* of the Applicant, or by an *agent* of the Applicant, or by *court order*, *and* the Applicant has no power to compel trust distributions.

❑ The value of a "work-related" annuity (pension, profit-sharing, non-qualified deferred compensation, 401k, SEP or Keogh) may be deemed unavailable for eligibility purposes if the Applicant has no right to require a lump-sum distribution; *e.g.*, a vested monthly benefit the payment of which commences at normal retirement age.

❑ IRAs are deemed unavailable if minimum distributions are being taken.41 They are also beyond the reach of DHS for benefits recovery.

❑ The classification of *commercial* annuities as unavailable is now fully developed. It began with *Transmittal 64* providing the federal view. The California view was published in *All Medi-Cal Eligibility Procedures Manual Letter Number 159*. ("Rules")42 Medi-Cal is required by the Rules to analyze annuities as "available" or "deemed *un*available" in four sequential steps:

❑ The *definition* of an annuity applies if the contract was purchased with "property of the applicant/beneficiary or spouse" after August 11, 1993 (the date the *Omnibus Budget Reconciliation Act of 1993* was signed).

❑ If payments are deferred because the Applicant or spouse is not receiving, or has not taken steps to receive, periodic payments of principal and interest, the cash surrender value of the annuity is considered "available" and the inquiry stops at that point.

❑ If the Applicant or spouse takes steps to withdraw principal and interest, but does not thereby (a) withdraw at a rate designed to "exhaust any balance" of the cost basis by the date on which his or her life expectancy expires, *and* (b) if the Applicant or spouse does not give up the right to surrender the contract (as is the case when exchanged for an immediate annuity), the contract is "deemed available."

❑ The life expectancy figure to be applied is taken from Medicaid's *Transmittal Number 64* (included in the Rules). The *Transmittal 64* tables are based on shorter life expectancies than are those in common use by commercial annuity carriers. Any payments to be made *after* the *Transmittal 64* expectancy period are considered a "transfer of property" which may be a *disqualifying* transfer. This could also happen with a period certain feature (*e.g.*, annuity with a guaranteed minimum period that exceeds life expectancy). Such annuities are described as "not properly annuitized."

Finally, if no disqualifying transfer is found, the Rules still require regular periodic payments, either in a fixed amount or in a fixed amount adjusted for inflation at a rate not to exceed 5% annually. If the installments do not meet this final test, they are considered "deferred" and the cash surrender value is considered "available." Apparently, if there *is* no cash surrender value, there is no down side.

3.7 Permitted Asset Transfers, Penalty Period.

Asset transfers must comply with the following rules:

❑ The gift of non-exempt assets to anyone other than an Individual's Spouse or a Community Spouse will start a period of Medi-Cal ineligibility (Penalty Period) precluding the Applicant's eligibility for up to 30 months (California never adopted the Medicaid 36-month look-back), or 60 months if transferred directly from a trust to the donee, following the date of the gift.[43] Subject to an exception discussed below, the spouse may not receive a gift from the Applicant then give it to someone else (such as the children) without incurring a Penalty Period for the Applicant.[44]

In a related area, if (1) the Applicant spouse is institutionalized at the time of transfer, or if (2) only property of the Community Spouse (not that received by gift from the institutionalized Applicant) is transferred, the Community Spouse may make gifts of otherwise-counted resources without incurring a Penalty Period for the Applicant.[45] To state the converse for clarity, if the Community Spouse receives assets from the Applicant and gives them away prior to institutionalization, a Penalty Period will be incurred. The reason is found in a differentiation between the DHS' classification of the Community Spouse as either a "Community Spouse" or the "Individual's Spouse." If they wait until one of them becomes institutionalized, the other becomes a "Community Spouse." A transfer of counted assets from an institutionalized spouse to a Community Spouse which is then given away to third persons does not cause a Penalty Period.

❑ The Penalty Period is calculated by dividing the state-wide average private pay rates for nursing homes into the value of the gift.[46] The state-wide average figure is announced each year by the Eligibility Branch of DHS, around February.

The Penalty Period runs from the first day of the month in which the transfer is made. Moreover, the fraction resulting from the Penalty Period calculation is rounded down to the next lower whole month under the rule that if an applicant is eligible for a single day, he or she is eligible for the month.47

❑ Property may be freely given by the Applicant to the Community Spouse, even if the value of the gifts exceed the Community Spouse Resource Allowance.48   It is the *excess* over that allowance that may bar eligibility, so the excess must then be redeployed (usually to an exempt or "deemed unavailable" category) or the Community Spouse Resource Allowance must be increased. The Community Spouse Resource Allowance may be increased by means of a fair hearing if the available income falls short of the Minimum Monthly Maintenance Needs Allowance.49

❑ The gift of property that is classified as exempt for Medi-Cal eligibility purposes may be made before or after application without effect on eligibility, because it cannot be deemed "made for the purpose of qualifying" for Medi-Cal since it is not counted anyway.50 That same logic applies to assets not counted because they are "deemed unavailable" to the applicant.

❏ *The Kennedy-Kassebaum Bill* was passed in 1996, effective in January 1997. Section 217 purportedly criminalizes asset transfers that bring about a Penalty Period. Often referred to as the "Granny Goes to Jail" law, this legislation upset many estate planners, perhaps because attorneys are to receive cells adjoining those of the offending clients.

The section is found in the fraud provisions of federal Medicaid law, and requires two elements: (1) an asset transfer that (2) incurs a Penalty Period. A less obvious element surfaced in time: it is aimed at people who hide assets to qualify for Medicaid, then *lie* about it.

The only asset transfer that incurs a Penalty Period is the transfer of a *counted resource* as a gift or bargain-sale. Such assets are generally cash, securities and real estate other than the applicant's home. As noted above, the gift of an *exempt asset* (home, furnishings, automobile, and others) will not bring about a Penalty Period, nor will the transfer of assets "*deemed unavailable*" to the applicant. Most plans are carried out without Penalty Periods.

Where the most desirable plan *will* incur a Penalty Period, at least two other options may be available: convert the counted asset to one not counted (exempt or deemed unavailable) *then* make the gift; or make the gift and wait for the Penalty Period to expire before applying for Medi-Cal benefits.

The second choice offers less certainty under the terms of Section 217. That is because the law is unclear about whether it is given effect (1) if the Penalty Period has expired, or (2) if the applicant waits until the 30-month look-back period has expired so Medi-Cal cannot even *ask* about the gift.

DHS has now implemented Section 217 in California by means of an *All County Welfare Directors Letter*. It will refer for criminal prosecution *only* matters meeting the following conditions:

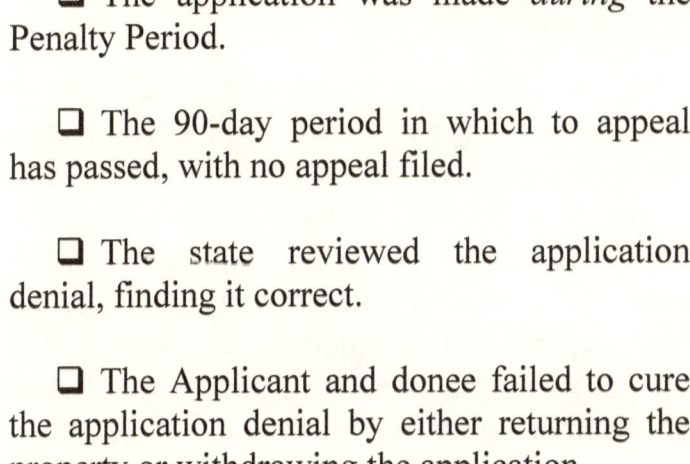

❑ The application was made *during* the Penalty Period.

❑ The 90-day period in which to appeal has passed, with no appeal filed.

❑ The state reviewed the application denial, finding it correct.

❑ The Applicant and donee failed to cure the application denial by either returning the property or withdrawing the application.

In this area, federal law proposes and state law disposes. The position taken by the state addresses the key ambiguities in a rational fashion. This is especially helpful in connection with the question of when the Applicant may safely apply. Now we know that all we need do is wait until the Penalty Period expires before applying for Medi-Cal.

Bar associations and other interest groups are working hard to have Section 217 clarified or repealed at the federal level. Until then, we simply follow state law and exercise sensitivity to this issue in designing plans.

3.8 Court Authorization for Plan Transfers.

Often, the lawyer is called after the Applicant becomes incompetent. Lacking legal capacity, *someone else* must act on his or her behalf in making the property transfers involved in the eligibility planning. If the Applicant had the foresight to sign a durable power of attorney for property that includes such powers, the planning may be carried out under its authority and without court involvement. More often, the power of attorney is inadequate for the purpose, either because the powers are not provided at all, or (given the narrow construction given such instruments by the courts) because they are too limited to be useful. We must then ask the probate court for the county in which the Applicant resides to substitute its judgment for that of the Applicant.

If the Applicant is married and the Community Spouse is willing to act as petitioner, the court orders may be obtained without the need for a probate conservatorship.[51] If the Applicant is *not* married, however, such orders are available only if a conservatorship is first established.[52]

Seeking such orders is expensive and time-consuming, especially for the *unmarried* Applicant. If obtained in a single hearing, the process may take as few as six weeks. You may succeed in combining a petition for appointment of the conservatorship of the person and estate with the substituted judgment petition and a petition to terminate the (newly-created) conservatorship of the estate (leaving only the conservatorship of the person). The procedural complexity, however, causes some courts to deny all except the petition for appointment of a conservator, requiring the other petitions to follow separately. That stretches the process out over months. Considering the added attorney time and the costs of long term care in that interim (because we cannot apply for Medi-Cal until the asset redeployment takes place, which cannot happen until the court authorizes it), such delays are unjustified from the standpoint of both the judicious use of court resources and the cost to the Applicant.

Added to the time and costs described above are those associated with legislative and judicial concern for the protection of the Applicant from artful and designing persons.

The court will invariably appoint independent counsel from a rotating panel. That attorney will meet with the Applicant and the family, examine the petition, consider whether the proposed plan is for the best interests of the Applicant (as opposed to the interests of the others involved), and report to the court accordingly. At the hearing, the independent counsel will inform the court of the time so spent and his or her usual hourly rate. The court will then order the fee paid from the assets of the Applicant. If there is no cash to cover that cost, the court may order it paid (at a much reduced rate) by the county.

Most of the time, a careful explanation of the rationale behind the plan will gain the support of the independent counsel. Occasionally, however, that attorney may have a personal or political agenda, or a faulty understanding of the related law, either of which makes it impossible to gain that support. The court relies heavily on the opinion of the independent counsel, but the battle can be won by presenting a well thought-out plan.

Generally, procuring the court's substituted judgment will double the charges of the planning attorney and add $1,500 to $3,500 for court costs and independent counsel fees. On the grand scale of things, however, the total is usually minuscule as a percentage of the assets saved.

Aside from needing court authorization for asset transfers by the incompetent Applicant, we must often seek other orders. Those other orders include increases in the Community Spouse Resource Allowance and the Minimum Monthly Maintenance Needs Allowance. They may be obtained from either the local probate court or an administrative law judge employed by DHS. The state will object to any order increasing the Minimum Monthly Maintenance Needs Allowance unless it is obtained through its administrative law judge, claiming that only *its* judges are authorized to make such orders. The state is incorrect, but careful wording of the probate court order is necessary in order to make the point. The income of the Applicant is allocated between the Personal Needs Allowance of the Applicant, private insurance premiums, Minimum Monthly Maintenance Needs Allowance of the Community Spouse and (the balance) to Share of Cost. It is undisputed that the probate court may order an allocation to be enforced against the Applicant. So the order should be drafted substantially as follows:

> "A Community Spouse monthly income allowance of $[   ] is established for Petitioner to be enforced against the monthly income of Respondent to the extent that Petitioner's income is inadequate."

I will spare you the details of pleading requirements and a myriad of factual and mathematical models, and instead move on to a discussion of the Special Needs Trust.

3.9 The Special Needs Trust

Generically, a Special Needs Trust (SNT) is simply one in which the trustee has sole discretion to determine the needs of the beneficiary and make the appropriate distributions from the trust. The discretion is governed by an objective external standard, typically the "reasonable needs" of the beneficiary for "care, support, maintenance and education." The discretion is further limited by the requirement that the trustee ascertain all other resources available to the beneficiary, including Medi-Cal, and that trust distributions will be made only to the extent those other resources prove insufficient.

There are at least two kinds of SNTs: those sanctioned by *California Probate Code* Sections 3600 *et sequitur* (Statutory SNT) and all the others (Non-Statutory SNT). Those sanctioned by the code most often arise from the settlement of a personal injury or medical malpractice claim where the estimated lifetime costs for special medical needs are expected to exhaust the net recovery. The deal with the state under a Statutory SNT is that (assuming no other disqualifying assets are owned by or available to the injured party) Medi-Cal eligibility is provided by not counting the net settlement reposing in the trust. On death of the Applicant-injured party, however, the state is entitled to recover from the trust estate all benefits paid or the remaining trust estate, whichever is less.

In determining the "net settlement," however, any amounts *then* owed to Medi-Cal are paid from the settlement, so the Applicant-injured party starts the Statutory SNT with a clean slate. Well, perhaps *almost* clean: the Medi-Cal right to reimbursement is limited to one-half the settlement, net after attorney's fees and costs.

If the Applicant-injured party recovering a settlement or judgment in a personal injury or medical malpractice action thinks the net settlement will *not* be exhausted by the costs of care, he or she will ordinarily pay any balance owed to Medi-Cal at the time the case is settled, leave the program (returning to private pay status), and use the trust to provide both special medical needs and *support*. Because the Applicant established the trust from personal resources (the settlement) and for his personal benefit, it is deemed available and eliminates Medi-Cal eligibility. However, if the estimate turns out to be incorrect, and the expenses one day threaten to exhaust the trust estate, it may be converted to a Statutory SNT in order to again qualify for Medi-Cal.[53]

If the Non-Statutory SNT is established by the Applicant, by the spouse of the Applicant, by an agent acting on behalf of the Applicant, or by court order, the trust estate is deemed available to the Applicant, precluding eligibility for Medi-Cal. That tells us that the Applicant funding the trust with a personal injury or medical malpractice recovery has two choices: put it all in a Statutory SNT so as to shift medical costs to Medi-Cal, and pay for therapy and training from the SNT; or put it in a Non-Statutory SNT, with Medi-Cal eligibility deferred until such time as the outside assets are spent down to $2,000.

For all others (the vast majority of cases), the OBRA limitations listed above are simply reversed-engineered. Well-motivated children do not wish to take the Applicant-disabled parent's assets and leave that parent on welfare; rather, they want to take whatever steps are necessary and reasonable to establish and maintain lifetime security for that parent. So when the parent proposes to transfer assets in the manner described earlier in this chapter, the children will ordinarily choose to use those gifts for the parent's benefit. The most reliable way to accomplish that end is for the children -- not the parent -- to establish a Non-Statutory Special Needs Trust for the benefit of that parent, funding the trust with (or from) the donated assets and usually serving as co-trustees. The trust is not created *by* the Applicant, or by the *spouse* of the Applicant, or by an *agent* of the applicant, or by *court order*. Therefore, the trust estate is not deemed available to the Applicant. The only Penalty Period or other restrictions on eligibility arise from the gift of assets, not from the existence of the trust.

The family must understand certain tax and accounting matters related to Medi-Cal eligibility planning and the use of special needs trusts. Those are discussed in detail at Chapter Four.

3.10 State Benefits Payment Recovery

On July 11, 1994, DHS made the changes in state law needed to comply with OBRA. [54]

The state *must* now "claim against the estate of the [deceased Applicant], or against any recipient of the property of that decedent by distribution or survival." Its claim is "an amount equal to the payments for the health care received or the value of the property received by any recipient from the decedent, whichever is less."[55] The payments for which recovery is allowed is the total paid for nursing home expenses and post-age-55 expenses *other* than long term care.

Recovery is mandated in similar fashion against the estate or recipients of property from the deceased *spouse* of a Medi-Cal beneficiary, at least to the extent property was transferred from the beneficiary to that spouse.[56] This provision has no authorizing provision under federal law, so its enforceability is in question for now.

The term "estate" includes probate assets, self-settled trust assets, joint tenancy assets, life estates and (presumably) pay-on-death bank accounts.[57] This tells us that retained interests in the gifts must be carefully characterized in order to avoid the reach of this rule. The most common retained interest is a reserved right to occupy the residence rent-free. This right is personal to the Applicant-donor, so it rises to the level of a general power of appointment, but not to that of a life estate. (A life estate also entitles the holder to all "rents, issues and profits" from the property, and may be sold or otherwise made available to creditors.) Therefore, the personal right to occupy underscores the exempt classification of the property (intent to return) while placing it beyond the reach of the DHS Estate Recovery Department.

The state must be given notice when a Medi-Cal beneficiary dies. Following is the form of notice my office provides:

> State of California
> Department of Health Services
> P. O. Box 2471
> Sacramento, CA 95812-2471
>
> Re: *[Name of Decedent], Deceased*
> Date of Death: [Date]
> Social Security Number [ ]
>
> Dear Sir or Madam:
>
> This firm represents the estate of the above-named decedent. [He/She] was a participant of the Medi-Cal program.

This letter serves as notice of death as provided by *Probate Code* §215. A photocopy of the *Certificate of Death* is enclosed.

Please notify this office whether there is a claim pending.

Thank you for your attention to this matter.

Very truly yours,

If a claim is made, a letter explaining the transfers and citing supporting authority is provided. Even though the matter is referred to the California Attorney General for review and possible prosecution, the well-developed eligibility plan leaves no opportunity for recovery.

3.11 Planning Possibilities

There are eight common fact situations around which most eligibility plans are developed. They are identified from the following questions and addressed by the documents listed for each:

Planning Issues

(Presumes Applicant Requires Long-Term Care)

3.11(a) Is the Applicant married?

3.11(b) Is the Applicant competent?

3.11(c) If married, is the Community Spouse disabled?

3.11(d) If married, is the Community Spouse incompetent?

3.11(e) Does the Applicant have children?

3.11(f) Are the children adult, competent and involved?

3.11(g) Can all assets be redeployed into exempt categories?

3.11(h) If unmarried, will remaining non-exempt resources exceed the Applicant's Property Reserve?

3.11(i) If married, do combined remaining non-exempt resources exceed the Community Spouse Resource Allowance?

3.11(j) If married, and combined non-exempt resources exceed the Community Spouse Resource Allowance, does the income of the Community Spouse fall below the Minimum Monthly Maintenance Needs Allowance?

3.11(k) Is the Applicant a Medi-Cal participant who is about to receive a personal injury recovery?

Document Assembly

The answers to these *Planning Issues* drive the selection of documents as follows:

3.11(l) If (a) is "no," (b), (e), (f) and (g) are "yes," and the others are not applicable, then we have *an unmarried, competent applicant with adult children who care, and assets which are exempt or can be fully redeployed to exempt categories.* We then prepare the following documents:

- Durable Power of Attorney for Health Care.
- Conveyance and assignment instruments for the gift of all assets to the children and over to the SNT.
- Special Needs Trust.
- Application for federal TIN for the trust.
- Plan Memorandum.
- Instructions to SNT Trustee.

- Engagement Letter.

3.11(m) If (a), (b) and (h) are "no," (e), (f) and (g) are "yes" and the others are not applicable, then we have *an unmarried, incompetent adult, children who care and assets which are exempt or can be fully redeployed to exempt categories*. We then prepare the following documents:

- Citation and Petition for Conservatorship of the Person and Estate.
- Draft Inventory and Appraisement.
- Draft Plan of Care.
- Draft 2580 Petition.
- Special Needs Trust.
- Court Order on 2580 Petition.
- Application for federal TIN for the trust.
- Conveyance and assignment instruments for the gift of all assets from the conservatorship estate to the children then to the SNT.
- Plan Memorandum.
- Instructions to SNT Trustee.
- Engagement Letter.

3.11(n) If (a), (b) and (g) are "no," (e), (f) and (h) are "yes," and theothers are not applicable, then we have *an unmarried, incompetent adult, children who care and assets which exceed the Property Reserve after redeployment to exempt categories*. We then prepare the following documents:

- Citation and Petition for Conservatorship of the Person and Estate.
- Draft Inventory and Appraisement.
- Draft Plan of Care.
- Draft 2580 Petition.
- Special Needs Trust.
- Court Order on 2580 Petition.
- Application for federal TIN for the trust.
- Conveyance and assignment instruments for the gift of substantially all assets from the conservatorship estate to t he children and over to the SNT.
- Plan Memorandum.
- Instructions to SNT Trustee.
- Engagement Letter.

3.11(o) If (a), (b), (e), (f) and (g) are "yes," (c), (d) and (i) are "no," and the others are not applicable, then we have a *married applicant who is competent, and has a competent Community Spouse who is not in need of long-term nursing, adult children who care, assets which are exempt or may be redeployed to exempt categories, and whose Community Spouse Resource Allowance will not be exceeded by the transfers.* We then prepare the following documents:

- Durable Power of Attorney for Health Care for each spouse.
- Conveyance instruments and assignment documents for the gift
- of all assets to the Community Spouse.
- Grantor Trust for the Community Spouse.
- Application for federal TIN for the trust.
- Simple will for the Community Spouse.
- Simple will for the Disabled Spouse.
- Trust Administration Memorandum.
- Plan Memorandum.
- Engagement Letter.

3.11(p) If (a), (e), (f), and (g) are "yes," (b), (c), (d) and (i) are "no," and the others are not applicable, then we have *a married applicant who is incompetent, whose Community Spouse is competent and will not need long-term nursing, adult children who care, assets which are exempt or may be redeployed to exempt categories and whose assets in the hands of the Community Spouse will not exceed the*

Community Spouse Resource Allowance. We then prepare the following documents:

- Citation for 3101 Petition.
- Probate Code §3101 Petition.
- Declaration, 3101 Petition.
- Conveyance instruments and assignment documents for the gift of all assets to the Community Spouse, pursuant to (yet-to-be-obtained) order of court.
- Grantor Trust for the Community Spouse.
- Application for TIN for the trust.
- Durable Powers of Attorney for Health Care for each spouse.
- Will for the Community Spouse.
- Plan Memorandum.
- Engagement Letter.
- Order on 3101 Petition.
- Trust Administration Memorandum.

3.11(q) If (a), (b), (e), (f) and (g) are "yes," (c), (d) and (j) are "no," and the others are not applicable, then we have *a married applicant who is competent, whose Community Spouse is also competent and not in need of long-term nursing, adult children who care, some non-exempt resources that exceed the Community Spouse Resource Allowance and the*

Community Spouse's income is below the Minimum Monthly Maintenance Needs Allowance. We then prepare the following documents:

- Authorized Representative form.
- Fair Hearing Brief.
- Conveyance instruments and assignment documents for the transfer of all assets to the Community Spouse.
- Grantor Trust for the Community Spouse.
- Application for federal TIN for the trust.
- Durable Power of Attorney for Health Care for each spouse.
- Simple will for each spouse.
- Plan Memorandum.
- Engagement Letter.
- Trust Administration Memorandum.

3.11(r) If (a)-(g) are all "yes," (i) is "no," and the others are not applicable, then we have *a married couple who are both disabled and both in need of long-term nursing but are competent, adult children who care, assets which are exempt or may be redeployed to exempt categories leaving no non-exempt assets in excess of the Property Reserve.* We then prepare the following documents:

- Durable Power of Attorney for Health Care for each spouse.
- Conveyance instruments and assignment documents for thetransfer of all assets to the children.
- Conveyance instruments and assignment documents for the re-transfer of all assets to the children as co-trustees of the Special Needs Trust.
- Special Needs Trust
- Application for federal TIN for the trust.
- Instructions to SNT Trustee.
- Plan Memorandum.
- Engagement Letter.
- Simple Wills.

3.11(s) If (a)-(j) are all "no," and (k) is "yes," we have *a Medi-Cal participant who is about to receive a personal injury recovery which will terminate continuing eligibility unless the recovery is shunted into a Special Needs Trust*. We then prepare the following documents:

- Plan Memorandum.
- Proposed provisions for use in settlement agreement.

- Special Needs Trust (statutory or not, depending on expert forecast of special needs costs).
- Application for federal TIN for the trust.
- Instructions to SNT Trustee.
- Engagement Letter.
- Transmittal to attorney.

Just to make this discussion more useful, here is a sample plan memorandum for a simple case.

Memorandum

To: Emma Lou McGillicuddy

From: F. Bentley Mooney, Jr.

Date: 07/19/02

Re: _Medi-Cal Planning Strategy_

Facts

Personal. You are 70 years of age, in poor health and presently in need of long-term custodial care.

Assets. Your assets include a home, furnishings, an automobile and about $40,000 in bank balances. The home is encumbered for $7,000, worth approximately $140,000 and has a low cost basis. The furnishings and automobile are probably worth $20,000 to $30,000.

Family Support. The children are all competent adults and cooperating in resolving your health care and Medi-Cal eligibility planning needs.

Objectives. You wish to give the home, automobile and furnishings to the four children, and to apply for long-term care under Medi-Cal. Those four sons are united in their wish to assure you maximum economic security under the circumstances.

Strategy

Gift to Children. Give the house, furnishings and automobile to Burt,

David, Dan and Jerry, reserving the right to re-enter and re-occupy the house and live there rent-free any time you are able to leave the long term care facility.

Re-Gift to Trust. The boys stated that they do not want your property, preferring that it be used to maintain your economic security. They further inform me that they will use those gifts to establish a Special Needs Trust for your benefit. They will also serve as co-trustees. In that capacity, they will rent the home and invest the cash to produce income for your benefit.

Penalty Period

Because all but $2,000 of the cash is counted in determining your Medi-Cal eligibility, giving it away will keep you from being eligible for a certain period of time. Here is how that period is calculated:

❑ First, you subtract the $2,000 property reserve you are allowed to keep. (Since it is not counted in determining eligibility, there is no penalty for giving it away.

❑ Second, give the remaining $38,000 to the four sons ($9,500 each).

❑ Third, divide the statewide average private patient rate into the net gift for each son to determine the unadjusted period of ineligibility. The rate is $4,163 for 2001, so the result is 2.28 months. The four gifts lead to four penalty periods, *which run concurrently.*

❑ Fourth, under the rule, "if eligible for a day, you are eligible for the entire month," we drop the odd amount, leaving a two-month period of ineligibility.

❑Finally, the date of the gift is backed up to the first day of the month. So, if all our plan documents and instruments are signed on the 20th of the month, the gift is deemed made 20 days earlier, on the first of that same month. We start there in determining the first day on which you are eligible, and that is the day we file your application for Medi-Cal. In the meantime, the children pay your long term care costs from the trust.

The Special Needs Trust

Income Tax Implications. The trust is ordinarily a separate tax-paying entity. However, because the trust estate will revert to your children on your death, they are deemed to be the beneficial owners of the assets. Therefore, any income -- whether distributed for your benefit or retained -- is taxable to the children. The trust contains a provision allowing them (as co-trustees) to reimburse themselves for any such personal tax liability. The only operating cost is a one-time tax return preparation charge to report to IRS that all trust income, deductions and credits will be reported proportionally by the children.

Your reserved right to return and live in the home will secure a step-up in basis on your death. The adjusted basis will be the fair market value on that date, and will, to that extent, avoid capital gain taxes.

Estate Tax Implications. This reserved right to return and live in the home will also cause it to be included in your gross estate for federal estate tax purposes. However, you are given a tax exclusion sufficient to cover the entire estate, so there is no requirement of a tax return and no tax to pay.

Retention of Home. The home will not be sold during your lifetime, for at least three reasons:

❑ Sale during your lifetime will require another deed from you, releasing your reserved right to live there. Without it, the children as co-trustees cannot deliver marketable title to the buyer. If you provide that deed, the boys will owe capital gain taxes on the difference between what you paid for it and the net selling price.

❑ Rental of all or part of the house while you are in long term care permits a return on investment based on its *pre-tax value*, whereas selling and investing the amount left after taxes will yield less income. Keeping it is better.

❏ The trust agreement itself *requires* the co-trustees to retain the home as long as you live.

Application of Trust Income.   Trust income is accumulated and spent for house maintenance and those of your expenses that are *not* covered by Medi-Cal; *e.g.*, better quality medication than those on the approved list, reading material, day trips, massages, hair care, manicures, etc.   It is *not* part of your share of cost for long term care.

Conclusion

On your death, the Special Needs Trust terminates. Children will sell the home divide the remaining trust estate equally between themselves.

At bottom, (a) the rental income may be accumulated to meet your needs instead of being applied to your share of long term care costs, (b) you qualify for Medi-Cal upon completion of this engagement, expiration of the penalty period and your move to the long term care facility, (c) the home is retained for as long as you live, and (d) your lifetime economic security is preserved. As incidental additional benefits, a modest inheritance is preserved for your children, capital gains taxes are avoided on later sale of the home, and the state may not take the home to recover benefits paid.

[End of Illustration]

This illustration does not go into such exotica as increasing the Minimum Monthly Maintenance Needs Allowance or Community Spouse Resource Allowance, or the redeployment of assets into exempt and deemed unavailable categories. But it serves to convey the principal concepts.

It is possible to make the transfers without a Special Needs Trust, but doing so exposes the personal security of the Applicant to a number of unwarranted risks. For example, one or more children may not live up to their responsibility to care for the Applicant-parent, or the creditors of one or more children may take the property and thereby make support impossible, or a child could predecease the Applicant-parent, or (without the clear ground rules found in the trust) the economic security of the Applicant-parent could be jeopardized by mismanagement, or receipt of the gift without re-gifting it within the same calendar month could render a disabled child ineligible for SSI and Medi-Cal. The Applicant may not need an attorney to engineer gifts, but he or she certainly needs one in order to anticipate and protect against these life risks.

Chapter Four

Tax Issues

Summary: *In the usual fact situation, a gift tax may be incurred but will almost always be covered by the applicable exclusion amount. Capital gain taxes may be avoided or minimized. Estate taxes are usually a non-factor for those prospectively eligible for Medi-Cal. Property tax increases may be avoided.*

This chapter deals with an area central to almost all Medi-Cal eligibility planning engagements, but almost never discussed in ways useful to principals and practitioners alike. It should serve to both guide and stir debate, perchance to move the art toward ever more useful levels of service.

4.1 Introduction

There exists widespread difference of opinion among tax return preparers with regard to the gift, income and estate tax aspects of Medi-Cal eligibility planning, especially with regard to the taxation of Special Needs Trusts. Conceding that it is an art in which everyone is entitled to his or her professional opinion, this chapter presents mine.

4.2 Gift Tax

Whether or not an eligibility Penalty Period is incurred, the gift of property from the Applicant to anyone other than a spouse may be a *taxable* transfer for gift tax purposes. If so, the tax may be paid by using part of the *applicable exclusion amount.*[58] To the extent the credit is so applied, it is no longer available for satisfaction of the federal estate tax. That, however, is rarely a detriment because there will almost never be an estate large enough to be taxed at the Applicant's death.

If the assets are transferred from the Applicant to the Community Spouse, the unlimited marital deduction eliminates gift tax as a consideration; no part of the applicable exclusion amount is needed.

The Context.   Aside from gifts from one spouse to the other, the transfers are in two, sometimes three, steps: from a pre-existing living trust to the Applicant (to avoid the 60-month look-back), from the Applicant to the children, and from the children to an irrevocable Special Needs Trust created by the children for the Applicant. The Special Needs Trust must always represent the *voluntary action* of the children (or other donees); otherwise, they will be deemed (and properly so) to be acting as the *agent* of the Applicant. If so characterized, the trust estate will be counted in determining Medi-Cal eligibility. The terms of the trust require the trustees to determine whether and how much to pay for the support, medical and long term care needs of the Applicant, *after* first using all of his or her *other* resources.   "Other resources" specifically referenced are Medicare and Medi-Cal.   As payor of last resort, the trust preserves the capital so as to provide lifetime security for the Applicant. That, after all, is the only reason to undertake such an elegant plan. On death of the Applicant, the trust terminates and (usually) reverts to the children in equal shares. Sometimes special needs of a particular child are included in the Special Needs Trust, to become effective on death of the Applicant. On rarer occasions, grandchildren are named as remainder beneficiaries.

Gift Number 1. For tax purposes, we ignore transfers from a pre-existing living trust to the Applicant as settlor, since (as beneficial owner of the trust estate) the Applicant cannot make a gift to himself or herself.

The gift from the Applicant to the children may include cash, securities, tangible personal property and the home. As to the *cash, securities* and tangible personal property, and as to the *outright* gift of the home (*i.e.*, without reserving the right to return and live there rent-free), the Applicant gives up all "dominion and control." Thus, a federal gift tax return must be filed.

As to the *home*, the Applicant almost always reserves (in the deed) the right to live there rent-free. Doing so underscores the exempt nature of the asset for Medi-Cal eligibility purposes. As with the gift of cash, securities and tangible personal property (above), the gift is complete, but considered to be so by means of varying analyses. Thus, this is a taxable gift whether or not the right to occupy is reserved.

As to the reserved right to occupy, the *Treasury Regulations*[59] treat the gift of the home as "wholly incomplete" or "partially incomplete" (thus, non-taxable) if the donor also reserves the right to decide who would receive it *after* the initial donees, but as complete if no such power is reserved. We do not reserve any such power to control the home after the gift to the children, thus the gift is complete.

Similarly, another *Treasury Regulation*[60] provides that if the reserved interest is not "susceptible of measurement on the basis of generally accepted valuation principles, the gift tax is applicable to the entire value of the property subject to the gift." Since the reserved right to occupy is personal to the

Applicant, it has no value to anyone else; *e.g.*, the Applicant is not entitled to receive the rent if the home is leased to someone else while he or she resides in a long term care facility. As a result, there is no apparent way to value the right to occupy under generally accepted valuation principles.

Finally, the *Internal Revenue Code*[61] deals with gifts to certain family members (children included) subject to a reserved interest which is not a "qualified" interest. A qualified reserved interest is one under which the Applicant receives fixed periodic income at least annually which is a fixed percentage of the fair market value of the home. The reserved right to occupy is not a qualified interest, so its value is ignored in determining the amount to be taxed; *i.e.*, the entire gift is subject to gift tax.

In the first case (no reserved right to occupy), the gift tax annual exclusion applies ($10,000 per donee per year, adjusted for inflation after 1998). In the second case (right to occupy reserved), the donees receive a remainder interest subject to the donor's personal right to occupy; therefore, it is a gift of a *future* interest and not subject to the gift tax *annual* exclusion. In both cases, the applicable exclusion amount ($1 million after 2005) for gift and estate tax is available, so the only actual expense is the fee of the tax return preparer.

In both cases, the basis of the children in each gift asset is that of the Applicant.[62] "Basis" is generally the purchase price originally paid by the Applicant, often adjusted to reflect depreciation or the prior death of a spouse.[63] It is used to measure taxable gain for income tax purposes on later sale. That basis figure may also be reduced *after* the gift to the extent depreciation deductions are taken on the home as rental property.

Gift Number 2. The gift from the children to the trust includes the cash, securities, tangible personal property and real property received from the Applicant.

If the trust estate remaining at death of the Applicant reverts to the children (or other donees) who created the trust, and if the trustee powers are subject to an objective external standard,[64] the gift is one of a life estate. That life estate is valued using tables provided under the *Internal Revenue Code*[65] and constitutes a taxable "present interest" gift.[66] The remainder interest (gross value less the value of the life estate) is not treated as a gift because it is returned to the children on death of the Applicant.

If instead, the trust estate remaining at death of the Applicant goes to anyone *other* than the children who created the trust (*e.g.*, the grandchildren), there are several ripple effects:

❑ The *full* value of the property is subject to gift tax on transfer of the assets to the trust, rather than the present value of the life estate.

❑ A "taxable termination" may take place for generation-skipping transfer tax (GSTT) purposes at death of the Applicant *if* the right to occupy is reserved by the Applicant. (This may be avoided by allocating part of the GSTT exemption in the gift tax return.)

❑ It makes the trust a separate tax-paying entity for income tax purposes, taxed as either a simple or complex trust.[67] Details follow.

4.3 Income Taxation on the Home

Sale During Life of Applicant and Prior to Gift. The one-time exclusion of gain (up to $250,000) on sale of the primary residence is available only *to* the Applicant *and* (a) if sold prior to the gift, and (b) if the Applicant resided in the home for 24 or more of the 60 months preceding the sale.[68]

Sale During Life of Applicant and After Gift, Where Right to Occupy is *Not* Reserved. The sale of the home by the children (as donees or as trustees), after the gift but prior to the death of the Applicant, may lead to a capital gain tax. Their basis is that of the Applicant, so the capital gain tax is on the difference between that basis and the net sale price, adjusted for any depreciation taken as rental property.

Sale During Life of Applicant and After Gift, Where Right to Occupy *is* Reserved. If the right to occupy is reserved, the co-trustees must obtain from the Applicant a quitclaim of that right in order to deliver marketable title to the purchaser. That leads to the same tax result as above.

Sale After Death of Applicant, Where Right to Occupy *is* Reserved or There is Continued Occupancy. The home may receive a basis adjustment to its value on the date of the Applicant's death, if the sale is made *after* the death, if (a) a right to re-enter and re-occupy to live rent-free is reserved by the Applicant, *or* (b) the Applicant continues to live in the property without paying rent at fair market value.[69] Such a reserved interest leads to that result, even if the health of the Applicant does not allow the right to be actually used. This is because the retained interest causes the home to be included in the gross estate of the Applicant for federal estate tax purposes, even though no return or tax is due.

4.4 Income Taxation of the Trust

Taxation to Children. The assets of most Special Needs Trusts revert to the children-settlors on death of the Applicant. Because of the relatively short life expectancy of the Applicant and the fact that the reversion takes place at the Applicant's death as beneficiary, the reversionary interest will ordinarily lead to classification as a "grantor" trust under the *Internal Revenue Code* for income tax purposes.[70] If so, it is classified as a grantor trust for both income and principal purposes, because the children (as co-trustees) are able to control beneficial enjoyment of the trust, with or without an objective standard for the exercise of discretion. As such, they must report personally their portion of all trust income, deductions and credits.[71]

Simple or Complex Regime. Where the children establish the trust for the Applicant *and thereafter for others*, then name an independent trustee and give that trustee distribution discretion limited by an objective standard, the trust is taxed as a separate entity; *i.e.*, trust income generally is taxed to the Applicant if distributed and to the trust if retained. For details, see *Accounting for the Special Needs Trust* at Chapter Five.

4.5 Real Property Tax

The central area of concern with respect to real property tax is reassessment under *Proposition*

13. If reassessed at the date of the gift, the tax goes up. If reassessed at death of the Applicant, a supplemental tax will be imposed on later sale of the property, covering the gap period between the two dates. The means of avoiding reassessment is the *Parent-Child Exclusion* discussed below.

"*Proposition 13*." is a shorthand reference to legislation imposed on the California legislature by voter initiative in the 1970s, expressed as a supplement to the California Constitution, denoted *Article* XIIIA and codified as *California Revenue & Taxation Code*, Sections 60 *et sequitur*.

The article added to the constitution contains six sections: Section 1(a) limiting the tax rate to 1% of fair market value; Section 2(a) returning assessed values to those existing on March 1, 1975 with modifications only for subsequent changes in ownership and new construction; Section 3 limiting the ability of the state to enact alternative taxes; Section 4 limiting the ability of cities and counties to impose "special [alternative] taxes"; and other sections dealing with the foregoing in detail.

The *Revenue & Taxation Code* at Section 60 provides that a "change in ownership" means a transfer of a present interest in real property, including its beneficial use, which is substantially equal to the value of the ownership interest. Section 63 excludes from this definition all transfers between spouses (including those effective on death). Section 63.1 does the same for purchase and gift transfers between parents and children. Its only limitation is $1 million on the trended base-year value of real property *other than* the parent's residence. The relationships include stepparents and stepchildren, parents and sons/daughters in law, at least until the latter relationships are severed by death, dissolution of marriage or remarriage. These (parent-child) transfers may be effected through trusts, but not through other legal entities.

Section 61(f) and 62(e) provide that there is no change of ownership reassessment on the creation of a life estate, except as given effect at the expiration of the life estate if the remainder interest passes to someone not covered by the parent-child exclusion. Section 65.1 does the same thing for "undivided interests."

All the foregoing makes clear that a gift of real property from the Applicant-parent to a child or children, followed by a re-gift to a trust for the benefit of the parent (absent evidence of agency discussed earlier), and the ultimate reversion of that property from the trust back to the child or children, are all covered by the parent-child exclusion. Thus, *none* of the gift transfers contemplated by Medi-Cal eligibility planning should lead to reassessment and increased property taxes.

On the facts with which we are concerned in Medi-Cal eligibility planning, the children (as transferees) must *claim* the parent-child exclusion. The form of the transaction -- separately at each step in the gift process -- is a deed, a *Preliminary Change of Ownership Report* and the *Claim of Exclusion*. The deed will not be recorded by the county recorder unless the other papers are filed (or at least the *Preliminary Change of Ownership Report* is filed) with the county recorder.

Chapter Five

Accounting for the Special Needs Trust

Summary: *If the trust is classified as a grantor trust for income tax purposes, the children-settlors report all trust income, deductions and credits. If taxed as a simple or complex trust, distributions are taxed to the beneficiary and retained earnings are taxed to the trust.*

Although IRS almost never audits private trusts, that is no excuse for failing to establish, characterize and operate them properly. The long odds are small comfort to the trustee who becomes the statistic.

This chapter serves to acquaint you with the manner in which income of the Special Needs Trust is reported. If the details bog you down, just refer to the *Summary* above.

5.1 Introduction

As discussed earlier, the Special Needs Trust (variously "SNT" or simply "trust") is a *payor of last resort*, and the Applicant is the beneficiary. (In this discussion, "Applicant" or "beneficiary" or "Mom," as indicated by context.) The term "payor of last resort" means the trustee gets at the end of the line; *i.e.*, the SNT pays for only that portion of the support, medical and long term care needs of the beneficiary which remains after all other resources are exhausted. Private insurance, Medicare and Medi-Cal are specifically referenced. The Personal Needs Allowance ($35 per month withheld from the Applicant's income) is also applied before a distribution from the SNT. Medi-Cal pays 100% of those long term care costs which exceed the Applicant's Share of Cost, 100% of doctor and acute-care hospital costs, but only selected medications and almost *no* personal services (hair care, massage, day trips, reading material, tape deck, television, etc.). As a result, medicine *not* on the Medi-Cal approved list and all those other non-covered items are paid from the Personal Needs Allowance and SNT.

If the gifts to the children include any cash, securities or other resources counted in determining Medi-Cal eligibility, a Penalty Period may be incurred during which the Applicant is ineligible. In that case, the trust also pays the costs of long term care (net after applying Social Security and pension income) until that period expires and the application for Medi-Cal becomes timely.

With this sort of planning, the state cannot reach the Applicant's former assets for recovery of the benefits paid, the trust income from those assets need not be spent on the Applicant's Share of Cost, and the trust distributions are targeted in a way designed to preserve the economic security of the Applicant-beneficiary for life. Preservation of the estate for the family is a mere benefit by serendipity.

I generally recommend that the children (as co-trustees) engage a skilled trust accounting professional to keep the books and records and to undertake the tax reporting. In many instances, however, they do not follow that advice, or the professionals so engaged are uncertain about how to account for trust operations. This section deals with that subject.

5.2 Grantor Trust Classification and its Implications.

A grantor trust is one in which the settlor has (or settlors have) retained either economic benefits or a sufficient degree of control over the beneficial enjoyment to cause the settlor to be considered the "owner" of the trust assets for income tax purposes.[72] The same or similar economic benefits or control may be given to a beneficiary under the terms of the trust, in which case that beneficiary (instead of the settlor) is treated as the owner.[73]

If it is a grantor trust as to the *income* interest, all items of income, deduction and credit attributable to income earned by the trust assets are taxed to the owner as if the trust did not exist. Similarly, if it is a grantor trust with respect to the *principal*, all items of gain, loss and credit attributable to trust assets are taxed to the owner as if the trust did not exist.

The assets of most SNTs revert to the children-settlors on death of the Applicant. Because of the relatively short life expectancy of the Applicant and the fact that the reversion takes place at his or her death, the reversionary interest alone will usually lead to classification as a "grantor" trust for income tax purposes, with the children as "deemed owners" of the trust estate.[74]   Another section,[75] however, provides that a gift trust under which the children (as grantors) are able to control beneficial enjoyment of the trust -- whether directly or as trustees, and with or without an objective standard for the exercise of discretion -- causes the SNT to be classified as a grantor trust for both income and principal. As such, they must report personally their portion of all SNT income, gains, losses, deductions and credits.

The difference in the facts assumed in the following discussion of simple and complex trust accounting and taxation, compared with this one on grantor trust accounting and taxation is what happens on death of the Applicant as beneficiary. There, the trust estate remaining is left to people *other than* the children who created the SNT; in this one the trust estate *reverts* to the children who *created* the trust. *That* pattern leads to taxation as a *complex* trust; *this* one leads to taxation as a *grantor* trust. In my experience, virtually all SNTs created by children for a parent will revert to the children. Thus, the grantor trust rules will almost always apply.

Making calls to tax professionals from time to time, I find widely differing opinions on the applicable tax model for SNTs, ranging from a wide-eyed shrug to insistence on ignoring the obvious. The problem is that such trusts are almost never audited by IRS, so almost no one is proven wrong. Perhaps some tax professionals -- certainly *clients* scratching their collective heads over this issue -- may here find some welcome relief.

We will assume that the trust (1) is irrevocable, (2) is established by the children for Mom, with the trust estate coming back to the children on her death, (3) Mom's assumed age is 89, and (4) the children are in their 50s and 60s. The present value of that reversion is more than 70% of the trust estate.

The *Internal Revenue Code* tells us that if that reversionary interest is worth more than 5%, the children as holders of the reversionary right are deemed to own the SNT estate for income tax purposes.[76]

Most grantor trusts must report under the general trust requirements. The annual income reporting threshold is $600.[77] Grantor trusts deemed owned in their entirety (as is here the case) are reported in skeleton form; *i.e.*, the children as co-trustees merely note on the *Form 1041* that this is a grantor trust as to both principal and income, and identify the persons reporting the trust income, deductions and credits (themselves), then report their respective portions on *Form K-1*.[78] As to the California return, do the same on *Form 541*.

As a deemed wholly-owned grantor trust, its tax reporting year is the same as its deemed owners (the children); *i.e.*, the calendar year.[79]

The principal concern with respect to grantor trust classification is avoiding "disintermediation," a five-dollar word for the children being stuck with the income tax and no offsetting deduction or reimbursement. After all, here they are working hard to design and operate an elegant plan to provide Mom with lifetime economic security, and they wind up reaching into their pockets each year to pay the trust's income taxes. Many cannot afford that extra burden.

In taking a closer look at this issue, let us further assume for the sake of illustration:

❑ that interest and dividend income of the SNT is on the order of $5,000 per year;

❑ that rental income from Mom's former home produces another $12,000; and

❑ that a Penalty Period arising from the gifts made by Mom leaves the SNT paying her long term care costs of about $32,000 per year until she becomes eligible for long term care under Medi-Cal.

Those long term care costs may be deductible as medical expenses, *but only by Mom*; neither the children nor the SNT may deduct an expense which is the obligation of someone *else*. (As discussed in the following section, the "distribution deduction" is available only to complex and simple trusts, not grantor trusts.)

Another problem is that the rent is a non-deductible expense: if the renter is one of the children, that child is making non-deductible rent payments, part of which comes back as taxable net rental income.

We may scramble for a solution by having the tenant make a $12,000 non-deductible/non-taxable gift to Mom each year *in lieu* of rent, though that grossly mischaracterizes the transaction and violates the trustees' duty to make the property productive. There is no easy answer to this conundrum.

The $17,000 passive income received by the trust (and perhaps passed through for Mom's expenses), is reportable by the children equally, even though the long term care facility ends up with the money. They, however, are also entitled to any expenses of the trust as deductions, and that may help to some small extent; *i.e.*, they could charge for services as co-trustees. That, however, would be a wash transaction ($1,000 deduction taken against

$1,000 income with nothing left over to apply to the net trust income taxed to them).

The only remaining idea in the scrambling category, is to redeploy the trust investments into tax-exempt bonds. The income will maintain the same character in the hands of the children (as deemed owners), so its attribution will not affect their personal tax liability. They make lousy investments, though, and raise a compliance issue with respect to the *Prudent Investor Act*. (See Appendix B.)

Moving from scrambling to forward planning, there is a way to deal with the burden imposed on the children as settlors: just authorize the trustee to reimburse them. They are already stuck with the income and estate taxes: How much worse can it be? Following are the unedited distribution provisions from my SNT forms:

> "4. **Distributions During the Life of Beneficiary.** During the lifetime of Beneficiary, Trustees shall hold, manage and distribute the Trust Estate only as follows:

"A. Trustees may pay from income or principal, or both, to or for the benefit of **[Name of Disabled Party]** ("Beneficiary"), such portions thereof, at such time, and for such periods as Trustees shall determine in their sole discretion, such amounts as Trustees deem necessary for the reasonable care, support and maintenance of Beneficiary. Any income not so applied or distributed shall be added to principal. As provided both here and at Section 6C hereof, Trustees shall consider other sources of support available to Beneficiary, including funds provided by the State of California or the United States of America, or both, in determining whether to distribute income or principal, or either, for the care, support and maintenance of Beneficiary. Trust distributions shall be made only after full participation in such programs by Beneficiary.

"B. [Settlor/Settlors] [is/are] deemed to be the [owner/owners] of both principal and income of the Trust Estate for federal income tax purposes under *Internal Revenue Code* §673, and the Trust Estate will be included in the gross estate of [any] Settlor under *Internal Revenue Code* §2036(a) upon [his/her/their] death during the term hereof. [Settlor/Settlors] [is/are] therefore required to pay all income taxes incurred by the Trust Estate, and may be required to pay estate taxes on [his/her/their proportionate] interest therein. In order to relieve that burden, Trustee shall distribute to [each] Settlor, on or before April 15 of each calendar year during the term hereof, cash in a sum equal to the obligation of that Settlor for state and federal income tax on [his/her/his or her] attributed interest in the Trust Estate, and on demand of the personal representative of a settlor who predeceases Beneficiary, that portion of any estate tax incurred by the deceased settlor's estate and attributable to an interest in this Trust Estate."

"C. In the event the discretions herein provided to Trustees are determined by a court of competent jurisdiction to render Beneficiary ineligible for any local, state or federal program of medical assistance, training or cash grant, Trustees may, in their sole and absolute discretion, terminate this trust. Upon such termination, the Trust Estate shall go and be distributed to [*e.g.*, the heirs at law of Beneficiary, share and share alike/Settlors, share and share alike].

5.3 Complex Trust Classification and its Implications.

For purposes of this discussion, we will assume an independent trustee and that the remaining trust estate goes to grandchildren of Mom as the Applicant-beneficiary on her death, rather than to the children who created the trust. That pattern requires gift tax reporting when the assets are transferred to the trust because the children-transferors retain no reversionary interests and the trustee exercises its discretion subject to an objective standard ("reasonable needs for care, support, education and maintenance"). It also makes the trust a separate tax-paying entity, taxed as either a simple or complex trust.

Given our working assumptions (independent trustee, remainder to grandchildren), the SNT will be a "complex trust" for accounting and tax purposes. For comparison, a "simple trust" is one as to which:

❏ all fiduciary accounting income (FAI) is *required* to be distributed;

❏ there is no *actual* distribution of principal; and

❏ there is no distribution or setaside qualified for a charitable contribution.

Any variation from those rules makes it a "complex trust".[80]

Taxation of complex trust income is analyzed in several steps: first determine FAI, then Tentative Taxable Income (TTI), then Distributable Net Income (DNI), then Distribution Deductions (DD), then calculate the tax on income retained by the trust and on income distributed to or for the benefit of Mom as the beneficiary. Here are your working definitions:

❏ FAI is all interest, most dividends and capital gains (*if* the trust requires their allocation to income, otherwise, capital gains are allocated to principal). *Not* included in FAI (because added to principal) are *capital gains* (where allocated to income), *stock dividends* (where there was no cash option), *liquidating distributions*, and depletion/depreciation *reserves* created under the terms of the trust or at the trustee's discretion. Subtract allocated expenses, *net* expenses for TEI and charitable deductions, but do not subtract the trust's personal exemption.

❑ TTI is FAI without deductions, plus capital gains, less tax-exempt income (TEI), less allowed expense deductions, less the trust's personal exemption.

❑ *Direct* expenses (*e.g.*, rental property expenses) are allocated to income of the asset incurring them, and, unless otherwise provided by the trust agreement, *general* expenses (*e.g.*, fees, commissions) are allocated one-half to income and one-half to principal. Expenses proportionate to TEI and any charitable contributions are disallowed. To determine the disallowed portion, establish the proportion of total income represented by tax-exempt income or the charitable deduction; that portion of indirect expenses is disallowed.

❑ DNI comprises interest (including TEI), dividends (subject to the FAI exceptions noted above) and royalties, all as modified by trust terms for allocation to income and principal.[81] For discussion purposes, DNI is TTI plus the personal exemption,[82] plus TEI (net of disallowed portion of expenses), less any capital gains not allocated to income or actually distributed (simple trusts only) and less extraordinary dividends allocated to principal. Personal exemptions are $600 for probate estates, $300 for simple trusts and $100 for complex trusts.[83]

❑ DD is determined in two steps: for simple trusts it is the lesser of FAI or DNI versus the character of the income distributed; for complex trusts it is the lesser of DNI or *total distributions* versus the character of the income distributed. DD affects taxation of retained income to the trust, whereas DNI affects income distributed and taxed to the beneficiary.

❑ Tax allocations to beneficiaries of complex trusts require separate treatment of Tier 1 and Tier 2 beneficiaries. Tier 1 are those for whom distributions are *required*. Tier 2 are those for whom distributions are discretionary.

A complex trust distribution is deductible for trust income tax purposes only if it is either a required payment of income or "an amount properly paid or credited or required to be distributed for the taxable year."[84] Discretionary payments, as in SNTs, are deductible only if actually paid or credited.

As noted, there are limits on DD: the first cut is DNI and the second is character of the income. For example, no deduction is allowed for the distribution of tax-exempt interest income, because that would amount to "double-dipping"; *i.e.*, deductible to the trust but not taxed to the beneficiary.

Example. Our SNT has a single beneficiary, Mom. She was in long term care throughout 2000. A penalty period was incurred because of gifts to the children in January, rendering Mom ineligible for Medi-Cal for the first five months of 2000. She was approved for Medi-Cal long term care effective June 1, 2000, remaining so for the balance of the year.

For calendar-year 2000, the trust received gross rental income of $8,000, taxable interest of $3,000 and tax-exempt interest of $1,000. Mom received $12,245 in Social Security retirement benefits, $12,000 of which was paid to the long term care facility and $245 of which was deposited by the facility in her Personal Needs Allowance account after she qualified for Medi-Cal.

The same year, the trust distributed $12,000 to the long term care facility for the January-May period, net after application of Social Security retirement benefits to her costs of care and net after application of Medicare benefits for medical needs, $2,000 for property taxes and maintenance expenses for the rental property and $1,000 in miscellaneous expenses.

Because there is no requirement that FAI be distributed, and because principal was distributed, or either of the above, this is a complex trust for year 2000. Thus, trust accounting and taxation for complex trusts apply, rather than those for simple trusts.

FAI. The trust's FAI is $9,500 (rent, taxable interest and tax-exempt interest, less the property taxes and one-half the miscellaneous expenses).

TTI. The trust's TTI is $7,983.33. Here is how it is calculated:

❑ Direct rental property expenses of $2,000 are subtracted from rental income of 8,000 for net rental income of $6,000.

❑ Delete the tax-exempt income.

❑ From the income remaining, deduct the miscellaneous expenses allowed,: *i.e.*, the amount remaining *after* calculating the disallowed portion allocable to producing tax-exempt interest. That last one is TEI ($1,000) ÷ FAI ($9,500) x indirect miscellaneous expenses ($1,000) = disallowed portion ($83.33).[85]

❑ Finally, subtract the $100 personal exemption for complex trusts.

That makes it $12,000 income, less $1,000 tax-exempt income, less $2,000 direct expenses, less the adjusted miscellaneous indirect expenses of $916.67, less the $100 personal exemption, for TTI of $7,983.33.

DNI. The trust's DNI is $9,000. (TTI ($7,983.33) + personal exemption ($100) + net TEI ($916.67) - any capital gains allocated to income or actually distributed).

DD. The trust's DD is $8,183.33. (The lesser of DNI ($9,000) or total distributions ($12,000) versus net taxable income ($9,000 - $916.67) + personal exemption ($100).)[86] No deduction is allowed the trust for distribution of tax-exempt income, so the class-adjusted income limits DD to the net remaining plus personal exemption.

Taxable to Trust. Since all net income and some principal were distributed, and since no capital gains were earned and retained in the trust, nothing remains to be taxed to the trust. More precisely, subtracting DD ($8,183.33) from TTI ($7,983.33) leaves a negative value, the excess of which is lost as a deduction.

Taxable to Mom. Distributions carrying out taxable income to Mom are $8,083.33 for year 2000. This trust has no Tier 1 beneficiary (all distributions are at the discretion of the trustee: Mom is Tier 2. The Tier 2 tax is the lesser of total distributions ($12,000) or DNI ($9,000) versus character of the income ($9,000 - $916.67 = $8,083.33)

Subject to special provision for specific gifts of money or assets under the terms of the trust, all distributions (regardless of specific assets distributed) are presumed to carry out income.[87] (The "kickout principle.")[88] The distributed amounts are usually deemed to consist of *pro rata* portions of each type of income realized by the trust.[89]

Do you wonder why I recommend the engagement of a qualified trust accouting professional to back up the co-trustees?

Appendix A

Program Descriptions

MEDICARE

One day in the spring of 1965, a young businessman took a seat at the counter of a coffee shop on Los Angeles' Wilshire Boulevard, near MacArthur Park. He ordered lunch, then responded to the friendly overture of the elderly gentleman on his right. From the ensuing conversation came a story that touched the young man's heart.

The elderly gentleman and his wife had retired several years earlier after selling his wholesale food business. They were then debt-free, with more than $300,000 in the bank and looking forward to a long, carefree and dignified retirement. Soon after, however, his wife developed cancer and he, emphysema. She died a painful death four years later, just a year before this conversation took place. The elderly gentleman had several years left to him, but they would not be enjoyed at a dignified standard of living because only $10,000 was left of their resources after paying for his wife's medical care.

As the young man, steeped until that moment in libertarian dogma, watched the elderly gentleman shuffle in tiny steps toward the cashier, stopping every ten feet to catch his breath, he silently acknowledged an epiphany.

Until that day, he regarded the then-pending *Medicare Act* as a dangerous first step toward socialized medicine. But the insight brought about by that conversation added mature perspective. If one can do everything correctly, attain the "American Dream" and still be economically destroyed by life circumstances beyond human control, surely society should extend a helping hand. This writer is that young man.

Soon after that encounter, Medicare was enacted and signed into law by President Lyndon B. Johnson. It is a two-part federal health insurance program for aged and disabled persons. One qualifies by being over 65 or by being disabled. The amount of income, whether from work or from investments, is not considered in determining eligibility.

There are two parts to Medicare: hospital insurance (Part A) and supplemental medical insurance (Part B). Part A provides hospital room and board benefits, limited coverage for skilled and intermediate nursing care benefits, part-time home health services and hospice care. It is separately financed by Social Security payroll tax deductions deposited in the Federal Hospital Insurance Trust Fund. Medicare participants contribute their part of the costs through deductibles and co-payments paid directly to the health care provider. Part B is voluntary and provides physician's services, certain outpatient services, home health care, diagnostic tests and medical appliances. It is financed from monthly premiums, deductibles and coinsurance paid by the participants and by federal contributions.

Medicare is administered by the Health Care Financing Administration (HCF) and the Social Security Administration, both of which are part of the Department of Health and Human Services (DHSS). DHSS contracts with private insurance companies for processing of benefits payments. The health care service providers select the fiscal intermediaries (Blue Cross or Mutual of Omaha) for the administration of Part A benefits. Under Part B, those intermediaries are selected by DHSS.

Title IV of the *Balanced Budget Act of 1997* enacted dramatic changes to the Medicare program, including shifting home health services from Part A to Pat B, and creating a new "Medicare+Choice" program (also known as Medicare Part C). HCF contracts with managed care organizations (such as HMOs) called "Medicare+Choice Organizations" to provide Medicare-covered benefits to those beneficiaries who choose to enroll in them. As a general rule, their claims are processed through the Medicare+Choice Plan and not through the fiscal intermediaries.

The vast majority of those participating in Medicare Part A qualify by being over the age of 64 and entitled to Social Security, civil service or *Railroad Retirement Act* retirement or disability benefits. Other ways of becoming eligible include qualification under the *Qualified Disabled and Working Individual Program*, or by being afflicted with end-stage renal disease or be being transitional-eligible. You may continue to work and still be eligible. Eligibility requirements for Medicare Part B are the same as those for Part A, except that the participant must also be a resident of the United States and *either* (a) a citizen or (b) a lawfully admitted alien who has resided in the United States continuously for at least five years on the date of enrollment. Those who are not otherwise entitled to Medicare may be eligible to enroll voluntarily if at least 65 years of age and either U.S. citizens or legal aliens who have resided here for at least five years.[90] A dependent or survivor of someone entitled to Medicare benefits is also entitled if the dependent or survivor is at least 65 years old.

A Social Security disability beneficiary is eligible for Medicare 24 months after commencement of disability payments. (There is, however, a six-month waiting period for disability benefits, making this a 30-month period following onset of the disability.) Those covered include disabled workers of any age and disabled widows and widowers over age 49.

Except for companies with fewer than 20 employees, employers must offer employees over age 64 the same health insurance benefits offered to younger employees. Medicare benefits are secondary to such health insurance programs, notwithstanding any policy language by which the carrier attempts to reverse the primary-secondary status. An employee may reject the employer's plan and rely solely on Medicare, but the employer may not structure the employee benefits program in a way designed to encourage rejection. Medicare is also secondary to individual health Policies, whether issued separately or as part of other forms of coverage; *e.g.*, medical coverage under automobile insurance, homeowners or tenants package policies, workers' compensation, comprehensive general liability etc.

Medicare Part A, Hospital Insurance

Most who are over age 64 but not eligible for Medicare Part A (because not then entitled to cash benefits under Social Security or the Railroad Retirement Act) may enroll for Part A anyway if (a) they pay a monthly premium for the Part A coverage, and (b) if they are also enrolled for Part B coverage.

Part A is financed by a Hospital Insurance Tax (separate from the Social Security tax) imposed upon employers, employees and self-employed persons. Every worker covered by Social Security or the Railroad Retirement Act must contribute. Since Medicare Part A benefit coverage is compulsory, no one may opt out of paying the tax needed to finance it. Medicare beneficiaries themselves pay for the dramatically new and increased benefits.

Medicare does not cover all health care needs of the elderly and disabled, nor does it cover all of the costs for the care received. For example, it will not pay for those charges deemed to exceed what is "reasonable and necessary" for specified purposes.[91] This leads to the denial of many claims, but appeals are often successful.

Subject to the deductible and coinsurance payments required of each participant the following benefits are provided under Medicare Part A:

❏ The cost of inpatient hospital care for up to 90 days in each benefit period. A deductible ($768 in 1999) is paid for the first 60 days plus a coinsurance payment ($192 per day in 1999) for each day of hospitalization after 60. There are also 60 non-renewable lifetime reserve days with coinsurance payments ($384 per day in 1999). There are also restrictions on hospitalization for psychiatric care (lifetime limit of 150 days and others).

❏ The cost of post-hospital skilled nursing facility care for up to 100 days in each benefit period. You pay a coinsurance amount ($96 per day in 1999) after the first 20 days.

❏ The cost of 100 post-hospital or post-skilled nursing facility home health service visits for a particular illness made under a plan of treatment established by a physician, except that there is 20% cost-sharing payable for durable medical equipment. Additional coverage for home health care services which do not meet the Part A coverage criteria and visit limitations are available under Medical Insurance (Part B).

❑ The cost of hospice care for terminally ill patients.

Subject to an annual deductible of $100 and 20% coinsurance payments, the following benefits are provided under Medicare Part B:

❑ Physician and surgeon services, whether furnished in a hospital, clinic, office, home, or elsewhere.

❑ Home health care visits, if not covered under Part A. Durable medical equipment, with some cost-sharing.

❑ A variety of diagnostic, physical therapy, chiropractic and podiatry services.

❑ Prosthetic devices (other than dental) which replace all or part of the internal body organ, including replacement of those devices, as well as braces and artificial limbs.

❑ X-ray, radium and radioactive isotope therapy, including materials and services of technicians.

❑ Surgical dressings, splints, casts and other devices for fractures and dislocations.

❑ Limited ambulance services.

❑ Blood clotting factors for hemophilia patients and items related to its administration.

❑ Hospital services incident to a physician's services to an outpatient.

❑ Dental services other than those for the care, treatment, filling, removal or replacement of teeth or structures directly supporting teeth.

❑ Antigens (if prepared by a physician for a particular patient), pneumococcal vaccine and its administration, hepatitis B vaccine and its administration (if at high or intermediate risk of contracting the disease).

❑ Services of a certified mid-wife.

❑ Partial hospitalization services provided by a community mental health center or hospital outpatient department.

❑ Screening pap smear and pelvic exams, prostate cancer screening tests, annual screening mammography for all women age 40 and over (the part B deductible is waived), colorectal screening.

❑ Diabetes self-management benefits, bone mass measurements, the cost of injectable drug for the treatment of a bone fracture related to post-menopausal osteoporosis.

❑ Eyeglasses following cataract surgery.

❑ Certain services by nurse practitioners and clinical nurse specialists.

❑ Certain oral cancer drugs and immunosuppressive drug therapy.

❑ Lung and heart-lung transplants.

❑ Outpatient psychiatric treatment for mental, psychoneurotic and personality disorders, subject to coinsurance of 50% (instead of 20%).

Expenses *not* covered by Medicare

Medicare does not cover long term care at the custodial level, if that is the only level of care required by the patient. Care is considered custodial when it is primarily for the purpose of helping with daily living or meeting personal needs and could be provided by persons who have no professional skills or training.

As to *skilled* nursing facilities, Medicare pays *only* if:

❑ the skilled nursing facility is Medicare-certified;[92]

❑ the beneficiary was hospitalized for three consecutive days prior to entering the skilled nursing facility[93] (or within the 30 days prior to entering the skilled nursing facility, if for the same condition);

❑ the beneficiary needs skilled nursing or rehabilitation services *daily* (construed as five or six days a week);[94]

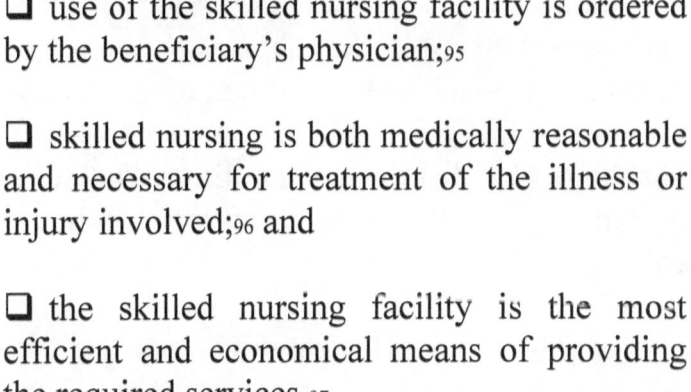

❏ use of the skilled nursing facility is ordered by the beneficiary's physician;[95]

❏ skilled nursing is both medically reasonable and necessary for treatment of the illness or injury involved;[96] and

❏ the skilled nursing facility is the most efficient and economical means of providing the required services.[97]

Medicare does not pay for services that are not reasonable and necessary for the diagnosis or treatment of an illness or injury. For example, drugs or devices that are not approved by the U.S. Food and Drug Administration (FDA), medical procedures and services performed using drugs or devices not approved by the FDA, and services (including drugs or devices) not considered safe and effective because they are experimental or investigational.

If a physician places a patient in an acute care hospital when a skilled nursing facility would be sufficient, Medicare will not pay for the excess over the cost of the skilled nursing facility because it is not "reasonable and necessary." Similarly, it stops paying when hospitalization is no longer "reasonable or necessary," even if the physician keeps the patient in the facility beyond that date. As you might imagine, this leads to a large number of challenges by disaffected families. The same notion applies to excessive office or house calls.

Unlike Medi-Cal, Medicare will not pay for services performed by close relatives of the patient. Nor will it pay for services paid by some other government program.

Doctors are not reimbursed for referrals to service providers the doctor owns (*e.g.*, clinical laboratory, physical therapy, etc.). The law prohibits a doctor who has a financial relationship with such a service provider from referring a patient.

In most cases, if the patient believed that a medical service or procedure was covered and it was not (*e.g.*, it was found to be unreasonable or unnecessary), a statutory "waiver of liability" prevents the health care provider from collecting the denied claim from the patient.

MediGap Insurance

More than 80% of those covered by Medicare *supplement* that coverage. Of that 80%, about 10% do so by qualifying for Medicaid (in California, Medi-Cal). The rest of that 80% insure those needs Medicare does not cover, or which it covers inadequately, through the use of "MediGap" policies. The function of such policies, as the name implies, is to cover risks Medicare does not insure, as well as deductibles and coinsurance requirements, thereby drastically reducing or eliminating out-of-pocket costs.

MEDICAID

Medicaid is a joint federal-state program of medical assistance to eligible needy persons, established along with Medicare in 1965. It is jointly funded and administered by the federal government and each state, plus Puerto Rico, Guam, the Virgin Islands and the Northern Mariana Islands.

Administrative responsibility on the federal side rests with the Department of Health and

Human Services (DHSS), which develops guidelines and supervises state and health care provider participation.

The federal government contributes approximately 50% of the program costs. The balance is funded by the states individually. Each state, however, exercises some control over costs by means of the discretion permitted in tailoring the Medicaid program for its resident participants. The states provide all local administration. In California, policy management and benefit recovery takes place at the state level and operations are delegated to each county welfare department.

Medicaid requires certain benefits be included in each state program, and authorizes others to be included at the option of the state. Thus, each state's Medicaid program is unique.

This discussion deals only with Medicaid, the federal program. A discussion of the California adaptation, Medi-Cal, follows. If you are not a California resident, you should consult your local welfare department for specific information about the coverage for your state or territory.

Eligibility Requirements

Medicaid is intended to benefit those who are eligible for Supplemental Security Income (SSI) and Aid to Families with Dependent Children, and who are financially needy according to program guidelines. In certain states, those who receive general assistance but do not qualify for SSI or Aid to Families with Dependent Children, may receive Medicaid benefits. The states are required by federal law to cover certain categories of people receiving public assistance.

Each state may choose between two arrangements for coverage of SSI recipients: it may treat every such person as eligible for Medicaid (SSI States) or it may establish more restrictive eligibility requirements for them as permitted by federal guidelines (Section 209(b) States). Section 209(b) States are so identified because the federal law permitting the more restrictive requirements is found at Section 209(b) of the 1972 amendments to the *Social Security Act*. Section 209(b) States may define eligibility for Medicaid more narrowly than the federal definition for SSI entitlement, or may set a higher minimum income level, or a lower maximum resources standard.

Because the rules that apply in California are of greater interest and utility than those from which they are derived at the federal level, we will just list the areas here and discuss them in more detail under Medi-Cal, following. Specifically, Medicaid sets the limits to be applied by the states as to: eligibility; asset transfers affecting eligibility; benefits; cost-sharing; recovery of benefits paid; appeals; and the rights of nursing home residents.

MEDI-CAL

California is an SSI State. It treats anyone who is eligible for Supplement Security Income as also eligible for its state Medicaid program, Medi-Cal.

Eligibility Requirements

❑ *Cash Grant Welfare Recipients.* Eligibility for Medi-Cal and all cash grant programs are determined at the same time, in the same process. Application may made at designated offices of the county welfare department. If someone is admitted to a county hospital and is eligible for Medi-Cal but has not yet filed an application, the county hospital will process the application on his or her behalf. On approval, Medi-Cal participation is established and it will pay the hospital directly. Cash grant programs include Aid to Families with Dependent Children (except for those over age 20 receiving state Aid to Families with Dependent Children, emergency assistance or unemployed parent cash grants), SSI and California's State Supplement Program, Entrant Cash Assistance, Refugee Cash

Assistance and In-Home Supportive Services. As a general rule, those under 21 who receive General Relief cash grant payments are eligible for Medi-Cal.

❑ *Certain People Ineligible for Welfare but Eligible for Medi-Cal.* Persons who are not able to qualify for cash grant programs may still be eligible for Medi-Cal. If the following requirements are satisfied, eligibility will be considered:

❑ over the age of 64 or under 21; *and*

❑ disabled; or

❑ blind; or

❑ a member of a family meeting federal Aid to Families with Dependent Children deprivation requirements; *or*

❑ pregnant; or

❑ receiving care in a skilled nursing or intermediate care facility; or

❏ a refugee or entrant who has been in the country less than 18 months.

Stated conversely, persons who are age 21 through 64 with limited resources, but who either do not qualify for a cash grant program or do not meet the requirements listed above, are not eligible for Medi-Cal benefits. Such persons (Medi-Cal Indigent Adults) may receive medical care from the hospitals and comprehensive health centers operated by the county.

❏ *Standing.* In addition to the foregoing, Medi-Cal eligibility requires that the applicant be a citizen of the United States or an alien lawfully admitted for permanent residence *and* a California resident.

❏ *Resource Limit.* Except as listed above, Medi-Cal eligibility is determined by the resources of the applicant. He or she may not have counted property valued in excess of $2,000 for a single applicant or $4,000 for a husband and wife as joint applicants. (Property Reserve) It represents the assets of the applicant remaining after deduction of all *exempt* assets and assets *"deemed unavailable."*

Exempt Assets

Assets classified as exempt, thus not counted in determining Medi-Cal eligibility, are listed generally in Chapter Three. To generalize even farther, it is usually the home, furnishings, an automobile, heirloom jewelry and prepaid funeral and burial arrangements.

Deemed Unavailable Assets

As discussed in Chapter Three, assets which are "deemed unavailable" to the applicant for Medi-Cal eligibility purposes, thus not considered, are those which cannot be reduced to cash within a reasonable period of time and those over which he or she has no control. In redeploying assets so as to bring about Medi-Cal eligibility, this is the second category to which we turn (exempt assets being first, and resource transfers with deferred eligibility last). See Chapter Three for a more complete discussion.

Income as a Consideration

Income is not considered in evaluating eligibility. It is, however, used to determine the applicant's share of long term care cost. (Share of Cost) To the extent the applicant has available income after subtracting enough to care for a spouse or dependents, unreimbursed medical expenses, personal needs allowance of $35 per month and perhaps home maintenance expenses, it is applied to his or her Share of Cost.

Two Ways to Receive Benefits

If approved for SSI or another cash grant program, or if approved for Medi-Cal with no Share of Cost (*i.e.*, no "countable income" to apply to medical expenses), there are two ways to receive Medi-Cal medical benefits: claim them either by means of monthly Medi-Cal cards, or by joining a health care plan. Those who *have* a Share of Cost will receive a Medi-Cal card only after paying, or agreeing to pay, for medical services equal to his or her share.

The Medi-Cal card is mailed monthly by DHS to program participants, other than those enrolled in a health care plan or who have a Share of Cost. The participant who is issued a Medi-Cal card may choose his or her own doctor, dentist, or drug store, being certain that they accept Medi-Cal patients. He or she may be required to make co-payments of $1 for most other services, including prescription medicines, unless under 18 years of age, over age 64, or pregnant more than one month. Co-payments may also be required for non-emergency use of emergency rooms. Certain medical services and prescription drugs not on the state's approved list require prior authorization from DHS in order to secure payment. The health care providers know which services require prior authorization, and will generally provide that service to the participant.

Those who receive Medi-Cal benefits through a local health care plan may select from a HMO, prepaid health plan or a primary case care management plan. In most cases, recipients will attend a state-sponsored lecture where the features are explained and the choice is made. Subject to certain exceptions, those using a health care plan must use its doctors, druggists and hospitals. With the health care plan, however, there are no co-payments, and the plan is not required to obtain prior authorization from the state before providing services.

Medical Expenses Incurred Before Applying

If medical expenses were incurred within three months prior to application for benefits, *and* if the Applicant was eligible at the time those pre-application expenses were incurred, *and* if the expenses incurred would have been covered by Medi-Cal if the Applicant had been a Medi-Cal participant at the time, Medi-Cal will pay them upon approval of the application.98 You must distinguish two related fact situations, however:

❑ Expenses incurred more than three months prior to the application for long term care benefits are *not* reimbursed; provided, however, that under *Hunt vs Kizer,* the Applicant may ask Medi-Cal to apply his or her share of cost to the satisfaction of unpaid medical bills which are less than four years old on the date of application.[99]

❑ Expenses paid from any other source will *not be reimbursed* by Medi-Cal. To be reimbursed, the health care provider must be persuaded to refund the money to the person who paid the charge; Medi-Cal will then reimburse the provider. Good luck.

Retroactive coverage requires a special form. You may obtain it from the Eligibility Worker to whom the long term care application is assigned.

Coverage While Out-of-State. Emergency care out-of-state is available. For information, the participant should contact an Eligibility Worker (direct-claim participants) or the health care plan in which enrolled.

Long Term Care Benefits. In addition to a full range of medical, hospital and skilled nursing care benefits, Medi-Cal provides long term skilled, intermediate and custodial nursing care, a benefit not found under Medicare. The following equipment, supplies and services are included in the Medi-Cal payment rates to long term care facilities:

Autoclaves.

Analgesics (non-legend).

Antiseptics.

Applicators.

Beds and bed rails.

Bedside utensils (*e.g.*, bedpans, basin, irrigating cans, drinking tubes).

Canes and crutches.

Charting supplies

Cradles.

Footboards.

Forceps.

Flashlights.

First aid supplies (*e.g.*, alcohol, iodine, bandages, etc.).

Gauze dressings, hypodermic syringes and needles.

Infrared lamps.

Irrigating standards.

Icebags.

Laxatives (non-legend).

Lubricants.

Mattresses.

Nail files.

Oxygen (all equipment necessary for the administration of oxygen other than nasal catheters and positive pressure apparatus).

Patient lifts and examining equipment.

Rubbing compounds.

Rubber goods (*e.g.*, rectal tubes, catheters, gavage, tubing, soft restraints, incontinence pads, urine bags, colostomy or iliostomy pouches and accessories.

Sterilizers.

Scissors.

rapeze bags.

Thermometers.

Tongue depressors.

Wheelchairs and walkers.

Weighing scales.

Other supplies and equipment used in providing intermediate and skilled nursing
care.

Certain supplies and equipment are *not* included in the Medi-Cal payments rates to nursing homes, but *are* covered Medi-Cal benefits. It is only necessary for the health care provider to bill Medi-Cal separately for them. Such separately-billed items include the following:

Drugs listed in *California Regulations*, Section 59999.

Physician-prescribed durable medical equipment which is custom-made or modified to meet a patient's special medical needs, which needs are expected to continue indefinitely.

Physician-prescribed prosthetic and orthotic devices for the exclusive use of the patient.

Allied health services which are provided by licensed or certified therapists and which are ordered by an attending physician (including without limitation, physical therapy, occupational therapy, speech therapy and audiology).

Medi-Cal participants must pay personally for the following items:

Beauty shop services (other than shaves or shampoos performed by the nursing home staff as part of patient care).

Cosmetics.

Denture cleaning.

Hair combs and brushes, personal laundry and dry cleaning, shaving soap and lotion, tooth brushes, toothpaste.

Television rental.
Tissue wipes for individual use.
Tobacco products and accessories.

In-Home Supportive Services.   Most frail elders and disabled persons prefer to live at home for as long as possible. Medi-Cal finds that less costly than long term care in a custodial facility, so to assist in that regard, so it provides in-home supportive services.

The services are, as you might imagine, provided in the home of the program participant.   They include both medical services and related non-medical services. The latter are aimed at enabling the participant to carry on the activities of daily living, and include personal care assistance (dressing and bathing), homemaker chores (cooking and house cleaning), nutrition and transportation.

The program is intended to benefit those who are eligible for SSI, and otherwise on a Share of Cost basis to those with modest resources but whose income exceeds the level required for SSI eligibility. The Applicant must also be covered by both Part A and Part B of Medicare.

Local community organizations (*e.g.*, adult day health-care centers, senior centers, congregate nutrition sites and transportation programs) are a valuable resource for in-home supportive services. Family members may participate by becoming caretakers and receiving minimum wage compensation from Medi-Cal for 40 hours per week. The service arrangements are designed by a case manager or case management team. Knowledgeable family members may serve in that capacity. Hospital discharge planners must provide some initial case management services for Medicare patients if asked by the patient or physician, or when the patient is likely to suffer adverse health consequences upon discharge if the planning is inadequate.

Professional case management is available on a private-pay basis. For those Applicants eligible for Medi-Cal, case management services may be obtained through the Multipurpose Senior Services Program if available in his or her county. Others may qualify for the "Linkages" case management program. Medicare home health benefits include "medical social services," which provide some case management functions in the form of counseling and assessment of financial and community resources.

State Recovery of Benefit Payments. The California Department of Health Services Recovery Unit is charged with the responsibility of recovering benefits paid to those participating in the Medi-Cal long term care and in-home supportive services programs. Recovery may be made from funds received by the participant, such as a personal injury settlement or inheritance, but most collections take place at the death of the participant. The authority is found in the federal Medicaid law.[99]

The recovery unit employs estate claims to recover benefits paid. Voluntary liens are used only if the heir or survivor agrees. If so, the heir or survivor of the deceased participant may remain in the property and the state collects only on his or her death. Voluntary liens are not recommended until the heir or survivor has exhausted all administrative and judicial remedies.

The second use of recovery liens comes about when an Applicant fails to state in the long term care application an intent to return to his or her home to live.[100] Unless the home is exempt under another rule, it is then counted in determining eligibility for long term care, and coverage is denied. To qualify for long term care while owning a non-exempt home, the Applicant must list the home for sale at the best price reasonably obtainable. The state then records its lien, and is reimbursed from escrow.

These are the only liens the state is permitted to place on the home of a long term care or in-home supportive services participant. Most often, the Applicant *does* indicate an intent to return, thereby establishing the exempt classification of the home. In that case -- if the home is not given away during life -- the state will file an estate claim after the death of the participant in order to recoup the benefits paid.

The benefits recoverable by the state by means of an estate claim are those paid for any Medi-Cal beneficiary to the extent paid after that participant's age 55, and all benefits paid to a long term care participant at any age, unless the participant is survived by a spouse or a minor, blind or disabled child.

The state is entitled to notice when a Medi-Cal participant or the surviving spouse of a Medi-Cal participant dies.[101]   The state is given four months after notice in which to file a claim against the estate.[102] If the claim is not filed in time, the state is barred from pursuing the matter.   The state may send the estate a questionnaire implying that the person giving notice is responsible for completing and returning the form. It is not required. All the state is entitled to receive is a notice and a certified copy of the *Death Certificate*.

The state may recover its benefit payments:

❑ from property owned by the deceased, directly or in trust, at the time of death;

❑ from property in which the deceased participant held a joint tenancy interest at the time of death;

❑ from property in which the deceased participant held a life estate at the time of death;

❑ The state cannot recover Medi-Cal benefits from the death benefit of a commercial annuity until it enacts regulations for that purpose. That has not yet taken place.

Unless property transfers are planned and executed with care and precision, the state may recover from the estate of the deceased spouse of the predeceased Medi-Cal participant. The property must be transferred from the participant to the Community Spouse in a manner evidencing a gift, so as to change its character to the separate property of the donee spouse. If managed in that manner, the state may not recover against the estate of the deceased Community Spouse.

The most effective way to avoid a recovery lien or claim is to adopt a plan that leaves the Medi-Cal participant with no assets. In a well-crafted plan, that will be the case.

Appendix B

THE PRUDENT INVESTOR ACT

The Prudent Investor Act became effective in California January 1, 1996. It is found in a section dealing with the duties of California trustees (*Probate Code* §16046).

The standard of care under *The Prudent Investor Act* is not based on risk alone, but rather on the appropriateness of the level of risk under all circumstances. Consistent with that, *The Restatement (Third) of Trusts (Prudent Investor Rule)* (1992), replicated virtually word for word in the California statute, flatly rejects case law and statutory approaches (often depression-influenced) which directly or indirectly resulted in restrictive lists of permissible investments, many of which provided levels of return so low that it was impossible to both generate substantial income and also protect the corpus from inflation. The new statute is designed to instead to compel trustees to analyze thoughtfully the trade-offs between risks and returns, taking into consideration the needs and objectives of the trust. The trustee should then consciously choose appropriate the level of portfolio risk and anticipated return.

The Prudent Investor Rule allows the trustee greater investment freedom than existed under prior law. For example, trustees were liable for portfolio losses even when the overall gains produced an acceptable total rate of return. Now, compliance with the new standards is judged as of the time an investment decision is made, not with the benefit of hindsight, leading to reduced liability for trustees.

One planning adjustment soon to become widespread is redefining "income" for purposes of distributions to income beneficiaries. By taking reasonable risks in order to enhance the total rate of return, rising markets will ordinarily lead to an emphasis on growth-oriented securities in the trust portfolio. The DNI (distributable net income) from a growth-oriented portfolio may be as low as 1% This works a hardship on income beneficiaries, while providing a windfall for remainder beneficiaries. To remedy that, the *Uniform*

Principal and Income Act now adopted in California allows trustees to declare some portion of trust receipts "income" and the rest "principal," with both tax and accounting effect. We use this power to substitute the following for the classic income distribution provision which simply distributes interest and dividends to the income beneficiary:

> Trustee shall add income to principal and from the common fund shall pay to the said [spouse/beneficiary] a sum equal to 4% of the Trust Estate value as that value existed on the last day of the preceding calendar year. Said distribution shall be characterized as *income* for trust accounting purposes, and shall be paid one-twelfth monthly or in other convenient installments.

Caution: a modified form is needed for income paid to a surviving spouse from a QTIP Trust.

Following is a specific investment policy statement for a balanced portfolio, generally suiting the needs of trusts having both older and younger beneficiaries:

Preamble

All funds of the trust are held by the trustee as a fiduciary. The following investment objectives, policies and directions ("the Policies") are to be judged and understood in light of that sense of stewardship.

Delegation

The trustee is authorized to retain one or more investment counselors ("Counselor") to assume the investment management of trust funds. In discharging this authority, the trustee shall receive reports from, pay compensation to and enter into agreements with the Counselor. The trustee may also grant exceptions to the Policies.

Objectives

The primary investment objective of the trustee is to preserve and protect trust assets by earning a total return appropriate in light of the time horizon, liquidity needs and risk tolerance applicable to trust distribution requirements.

Asset Allocation

To accomplish these investment objectives, the Counselor may be authorized to utilize portfolios of equity (common stock and convertible preferred), fixed-income securities and short-term investments. The Counselor shall observe the *Maximum Percentage Policies* described below, as modified from time to time by the trustee. The actual investment aims shall be set within those limits by the Counselor and trustee.

Maximum Percentage Policies per Investment Fund or Category

Investment Fund	Asset Classes		
	Equities	Fixed	Short-Term
Operating Reserves	0%	50%	100%
Long Term Funds	80%	50%	20%

Asset Quality

Common Stock. The quality rating for at least 50% of common stocks shall be B+ or better, as rated by Standard & Poor's or another equivalent rating service. The Counselor may use non-rated common stocks, at its discretion, within this guideline.

Convertible Preferred Stock and Convertible Bonds. Convertible preferred stock is permitted, but not straight preferred stock. The quality rating of convertible preferred and convertible bonds shall be BBB or better, as rated by Standard & Poor's, or Baa or better, as rated by Moody's. The common stock into which either may be converted shall be rated B+ or better, as rated by Standard & Poor's or another equivalent rating service.

Fixed-Income Securities. The quality rating of bonds and notes shall be A+BBB or better, as rated by Standard & Poor's or Moody's. The portfolio may consist of only traditional principal and interest obligations (no derivatives) with maturities of seven years or less.

Short-Term Reserves. The quality rating of commercial paper shall be A-1, as rated by Standard & Poor's, P-1, as rated by Moody's, or better. The assets of any money market mutual funds shall comply with the quality provisions for fixed-income securities or short-term reserves;

provided, however, that it is acknowledged that such funds may contain minor portions invested in derivatives for risk control.

Asset Diversification

As a general policy, the Counselor shall maintain reasonable diversification at all times. In that regard, the Counselor may not allow the investments in the equity securities of any one company to exceed 5% of the portfolio, nor the total securities position (debt and equity) in any one company to exceed 10% or the portfolio. The Counselor shall also maintain reasonable sector allocations and diversification. In that regard, no more than 25% of the entire portfolio may be invested in the securities of any one sector.

Transactions

All purchases of securities shall be for cash. Margin purchases are prohibited, as are short selling and commodity transactions.

[OPTION]
Moral Issues

It is the aim of the trustee to invest in companies the business conduct of which is consistent with family goals and beliefs. Therefore, the Counselor shall use its best efforts to avoid investing directly or through mutual funds in the securities of any company known to participate in businesses the family deems morally offensive.

[CONTINUE]

Reporting Requirements

Monthly. The Counselor shall provide the trustee with a monthly written report containing all pertinent transaction details for the preceding month, including:

❑ the name and quantity of each security purchased or sold, with the price and transaction date;

❑ an analysis for each security of its percentage of total portfolio, purchase date, quantity, average cost basis, current market value, unrealized gain or loss, and indicated annual income and yield at market; and

❑ an analysis for the entire portfolio of the current asset allocation by investment category.

Periodically. The Counselor shall meet with the trustee quarterly or semi-annually to provide detailed information about (a) asset allocation, (b) investment performance, (c) future investment strategies, and (d) any other matters of interest to the trustee.

Annually. The Counselor shall provide an annual summary of all transactions in each fiscal year, together with a report of investment performance for the year.

Cash Flow Requirements. The trustee shall be responsible for advising the Counselor in a timely manner of cash distribution requirements from any managed account. The Counselor is responsible for providing adequate liquidity in the accounts to meet the cash flow requirements so presented.

Glossary of Abbreviations

ACWD	All-County Welfare Directors' Letter
DD	Distribution deductions
DHS	California Department of Health Services
DHHS	(Federal) Department of Health and Human Services
DHS	(California) Department of Health Services
DNI	Distributable net income
DPAHC	Durable power of attorney for health care
FAI	Fiduciary accounting income
GSTT	Generation-Skipping Transfer Tax
HCFA	Health Care Financing Administration
HMO	Health maintenance organization
ILIT	Irrevocable Life Insurance Trust

IRA	Individual Retirement Account
IRC	Internal Revenue Code
IRD	Income in respect of a decedent
MCCA	Medicare Catastrophic Coverage Act of 1988
OBRA '87	Consolidated Omnibus Budget Reconciliation Act of 1987
OBRA '93	Consolidated Omnibus Budget Reconciliation Act of 1993
OID	Original issue discount
QTIP	Qualified Terminable Interest Property
Roth IRA	Roth Individual Retirement Account
RRA	Railroad Retirement Act
S/HMO	Social/Health Maintenance Organization
SNT	Special Needs Trust
SSI	Supplemental Security Income
TEI	Tax-exempt income
TTI	Tentative taxable income

Topical Index

Endnotes

[1] . *ACWD Letter* 93-63, *Policy and Procedures Manual,* Letter 242 dated April 23, 2001.

[2] . Reg 25.2503-2; *Commissioner vs Bowing* 123 F2d 86.

[3] . *Crummey vs Commissioner* 9th Cir (1968) 397 F2d 82.

[4] . *IRC* §2042; Reg 20.2042-1(c)(4); *Farwell vs U.S.*, 243 F2d 373; *In Re Rhodes*, 174 F2d 548; *Seward's Estate vs Commissioner*, 164 F2d 434.

[5] . *Rev Rul* 69-54, 1969-1 CB 221; se also *Rev Rul* 72-307, 1972-1 CB 307.

[6] . *IRC* §2035.

[7] . *IRC* §2035(c).

[8] . With applicants in less than perfect health, several questions arise in submitting an application:

❏ Who is likely to take this applicant, given his or her state of health?
❏ Who is going to give this applicant a preferred rate, or at least a standard rate?

❑ What are the chances of favorable underwriting from the first choice carrier?

❑ If the first carrier rejects, will this applicant be able to obtain coverage elsewhere?

A carrier that declines 40% of the applications received and raises the rates for half of the others may not be a good place to start if the applicant has a problem, such as diabetes, hypertension or congestive heart failure. It is important to use an agent who has this information and knows how to use it.

In 1998, StrateCision, Inc., a Needham, Massachusetts developer of sales and training software for long term care insurance agents, surveyed 35 of the major long term care carriers regarding their underwriting practices. It found first that such an inquiry is viewed with same reluctance as borrowing underwear.

20 of the 35 refused to disclose anything about their underwriting practices, even after being assured that only summary statistics would be published. This, apparently, is a closely-guarded trade secret. As to the others, they accept 47% of the applications received at their preferred rates, although the company-by-company variations ranged from 3% to 74% The necessary implication from this is that some carriers use the preferred rate as the norm, while others reserve it for those who fall from heaven with their pockets

full of manna. The variation was less with respect to the rejection rate. The average was 15%, and ranged from 8% to 25%, with most in the range of 13% to 20%

As to current trends, 26% thought underwriting was becoming more liberal, while 5% saw them as tighter. The others felt they were substantially unchanged. 32% opined that underwriting will be come easier on the applicant, while 5% expect it to be tougher. Again, the others foresee no change.

Looking at variation in current underwriting standards, using the underwriting guides of 23 larger long term care carriers, substantial uniformity is found in several areas. For example, applicants with AIDS, cirrhosis, multiple sclerosis, muscular dystrophy and Parkinson's Disease are routinely declined, whereas those with diabetes can be acceptable or uninsurable, depending on the type and the carrier. Knowing these differences at the time of application may make a difference between getting insured or getting rejected.

[9]. *Private Financing of Long-Tern Care: Current Methods and Resources,* ICF, Inc.

[10]. *The State of Long- Term Care Insurance,* Nov. 25, 1986.

[11]. *IRC* §408(a).

[12]. *IRC* §408A(a).

[13]. *IRC* §408A(c)(1).

[14]. *IRC* §408A(d)(3).

[15]. *IRC* §408A(d)(1).

[16]. *IRC* §408A(c)(4) and (5).

[17]. ACWDL #90-01, Question 3, provides for *no look-back period* when applying for coverage as medically indigent (such as SSI) or for In-Home Supportive Services. That means there is no Penalty Period for transferring assets in order to qualify for Medi-Cal. That changes, however, if the Applicant is institutionalized and seeks long term care coverage.

[18]. *All County Welfare Directors Letter (ACWD Letter)* 89-93; 42 *USC* 1396r-5(f).

[19]. 42 *USC* 1396r-5(b)(2).

[20]. 42 *USC* 1396r-5(c)(4); draft *Code of Regulations* §50490.3(e). Beginning with the calendar month after the Applicant is approved for long term care under Medi-Cal, any assets acquired by the

Community Spouse are not considered available to the

Applicant. Therefore, if the Community Spouse, for example, then receives an inheritance, it will have no effect on the continuing eligibility of the Applicant.

[21]. *Code of Regulations* §50701(c); *ACWD Letter* 90-01, Question 29.

[22]. 42 *USC* 1396r-5(b); (Draft) *Code of Regulations* §50512 attached to *ACWD Letter* 90-03 (January 8, 1990).

[23]. *Code of Regulations* §50605.

[24]. *Code of Regulations* §50425. The code section is the subject of certain ACWDLs, most recently Number 95-48. There, the Chief of the Medi-Cal Eligibility Branch made it abundantly clear to the county welfare directors:

❑ that the principal residence is exempt based on the Applicant's *subjective* intent to return, even though the *ability* to return may never exist;
❑ that the intent to return is indicated on the *Statement of Facts* (one of the Medi-Cal application forms for long term care) at Question 17A;
❑ that the county may not restrict the process of indicating the intent to return to the residence;

❑ that the county must not require *verification* of the Applicant's *ability* to return, unless the Applicant requests a deduction from Share of Cost for home maintenance expenses under *Code of Regulations* §50605; and

❑ that if the Applicant answers Question 17A indicating *no* intent to return and later expresses a wish to *change* that answer, *the county must accept that correction.* This last point is based on the fact that many do not understand the implication of stating no intent to return; *i.e.*, that it renders the residence non-exempt for Medi-Cal eligibility purposes.

25. *Code of Regulations* §50526.

26. August 3, 1990 *Department of Health Services Letter* Number 3, citing *Draft Code of Regulations* §50490.1 contained in *ACWD Letter* 90-01.

27. *Code of Regulations* §50461.

28. *Code of Regulations* §50465.

29. *Code of Regulations* §50467.

30. *Code of Regulations* §50469.

31. *Code of Regulations* §50471.

[32]. *Code of Regulations* §50476.

[33]. *Code of Regulations* §50479; *ACWD Letter* 93-71.

[34]. *Code of Regulations* §50477.

[35]. *Code of Regulations* §50485; *ACWD Letter* 95-22. From 1991 to 1995, practitioners relied on ACWDL #91-28 and draft Code of Regulations §50485(d) to shelter income-producing real estate. The regulation provides in relevant part, "...real property used in whole or in part as a business or as a means of self-support shall be exempt. On April 3, 1995, DHS issued ACWDL #95-22, to announce that, "... ACWDL #91-28 means self-employment rather than just an arrangement which provides financial support,...." The result is that DHS views real property used simply for "investment income" as non-exempt.

This position notwithstanding, the language of the code section is clear and unambiguous in classifying as exempt any and all income-producing real property held as an investment, whether or not it is tied to self-employment. Depending on the confidence of the practitioner and the willingness of the Applicant to press the issue, it should be worthwhile to assert in the application that the property is exempt, take the denial to an appeal and make that argument to an administrative law judge, asking for reversal of the county action.

[36]. *Code of Regulations* §50485.

[37]. *Code of Regulations* §50475.

[38]. Section 14006(c).

[39]. *Pub.L. Number* 100-203, 101 Stat. 1330.

[40]. *Pub.L. Number* 100-203, §9103.

[41]. *Code of Regulations* §50548(a), (e) and (f).

[42]. The Rules leave us with three different sources of authority on the Medi-Cal treatment of annuities: the original proposed regulations from December 1995, some undated state training materials entitled *Treatment of Trust and Annuities for Medi-Cal Eligibility*, and now the Rules. In addition, *Draft 22 CCR* §50402 on "availability" remains in effect, with continuing relevance for annuities not covered by the Rules.

[43]. 42 *USC* 1396p(c). The separate look-back rule for gifts made from the applicant's living trust is bizarre. It provides that the look-back period is 60

months "in the case of payments from a trust or portions of a trust that are treated as assets disposed of by the individual [to another person from a revocable trust established by the beneficiary or when a beneficiary settlor is foreclosed from receiving any benefits from an irrevocable trust]." What is the supposed purpose of giving this special attention to gifts made from the applicant-settlor's personal living trust, as opposed to the rule that applies if he or she first takes the property *out* of the trust *then* makes the gift? Silly, but easy enough to avoid.

44.   42 *USC* 1396r-5(f).

45.   *Draft Code of Regulations* §50411.5(a)(3); *ACWD Letter* 90-01.

46.   *ACWD Letter* 90-58.

47.   *Code of Regulations* §50701(c); *ACWD Letter* 90-01, Question 29.

48.   42 *USC* 1396r-5(f).

49.   42 *USC* 1396r-5(e)(A) and (C); *ACWD Letter* 90-01; *Draft Code of Regulations* §50490.5.

50.   *ACWD Letter* 90-01, Questions 7 and 8.

[51]. *Probate Code* §3101 *et seq.* Until 1996, *Probate Code* §3100 limited substituted judgment powers to community property. That year, subsection (b) was added to Section 3100 to allow the court to authorize the transfer of *separate* property. Section 3144(a)(1), however, was not changed and continues to reflect only community property transfers. Similarly, Section 3121(g) continues to require an allegation in the petition that the property is *community* property. This has all the earmarks of legislative oversight, so it must be brought to bring it to the court's attention in petitioning for these substituted judgment orders where some of the property involved is the separate property of the applicant.

[52]. *Probate Code* §2580 *et seq.*

[53]37. There is some debate about whether this is permitted under the *Probate Code*, and I frankly have a hard time understanding it myself. But an executive at the Department of Health Services informs me that they routinely approve such conversions. It does require a court order, and obtaining that order will be facilitated by drafting the trust in the first instance with this possibility in mind.

[54]. AB 2377, now Chapter 147, Statutes of 1994.

[55]. *Welfare & Institutions Code* §14009.5(a).

[56]. *Welfare & Institutions Code* §14005.9(b)(2)(A).

[57]. 42 *USC* 1396p(b)(4)(B).

[58]. *IRC* §2505.

[59]. *Treasury Regulation* 25.2511-2(b).

[60]. *Treasury Regulation* 25.2511-1(e).

[61]. *Internal Revenue Code* §2702.

[62]. *Internal Revenue Code* §1015.

[63]. Under *Internal Revenue Code* §1014, basis is adjusted to the date of death value on death of the owner. If a prior spouse held an interest in a marital asset on the date of death, its basis is adjusted in this manner. Whether the interest of the surviving spouse receives a concurrent adjustment turns on how title was held. If the property was held in joint tenancy, IRS views that as two separate property interests and allows a basis adjustment only for the decedent spouse's interest. If the property was held in community property title, however, it is seen as an undivided one-half interest in the whole, and the entire property receives a basis adjustment; *i.e.*, both the

interest of the deceased spouse *and* that of the surviving spouse.

[64]. For example, the "reasonable care, support, maintenance and education" of the beneficiary.

[65]8. Section 7520.

[66]. *Internal Revenue Code* §2511; Reg 25.2511-2(h)(7) and (g).

[67]. See the discussion of trust taxation, *infra*.

[68]. *Internal Revenue Code* §121; §1034 repealed).

[69]. *Internal Revenue Code* §§ 2036(a), 1014.

[70]. *Internal Revenue Code* §673.

[71]. *Internal Revenue Code* §674(a).

[72]. *IRC* §§673-677.

[73]. *IRC* §678.

[74]. *IRC* §673.

[75]. *IRC* §674(a).

[76]. *IRC* §673.

[77]. *IRC* §6012(a)(4).

[78]. Reg 1.671-4(a); instructions to IRS *Form 1041*).

[79]. *Rev Rul* 90-55, 1990-2 CB 161.

[80]. There is an exception for income in respect of a decedent (taxable to the trust but received as and allocated to principal); no distribution deduction available to the trust. There is also an exception for tax exempt income (included in FAI and distributable net income (DNI) per *IRC* §651(a)).

Section 651 deals with simple trust taxation. Section 652 deals with inclusions in beneficiary gross income.

Section 661 deals with complex trust taxation. Section 662 deals with inclusions in beneficiary gross income.

[81]. DNI may also include -- taxable but not necessarily distributable -- depreciation recapture, recapture of intangible drilling costs deductions, undistributed Subchapter-S corporation income, undistributed Subpart F income, Income in Respect of a Decedent (IRD) and imputed interest under the Original Issue Discount (OID) Rules.

82. *IRC* §643(b).

83. *Ibid.*

84. *IRC* §661.

85. *IRC* §265(a).

86. *IRC* §661(a)(1).

87. *Ibid.* But see Section 663 for certain exceptions.

88. On the issue of distributions carrying out income:

    (a) All *required* distributions of FAI are deemed distributions for Subchapter J purposes.

    (b) All *discretionary* distributions of FAI are distributions only if actually distributed.

    (c) All other distributions are deemed to carry out FAI except specific (non-income) specific gifts described at *IRC* §663(a)(1). They are:

        (1) Specific *sums* or specific *property*.

(2)   Paid or credited in three or fewer installments.

(3)   Based on the terms of the will or trust on: Date of Death (will); or on Date of Execution or Date it Becomes Irrevocable, whichever comes first (trust).

89.   *IRC* §661(b).

90.   42 *U.S.C.* 1395i-2(a), 1395o; 42 *CFR* 406.5(b), 406.20, 407.10.

91.   42 *U.S.C.* 1395y(a)(1); 42 *CFR* 411.15k.

92.   42 *USC* 1395i-3(a)(3), 1395cc(a)(1); 42 *CFR* 489.20.

93.   *Social Security Act* §1861(i); 42 *CFR* 409.30; *HCFA Medicare Intermediary Manual* §3131.3; *HCFA Skilled Nursing Manual* §212.1.

94.   42 *CFR* 409.34.

95.   42 *USC* 1395f(a)(2)(C); 42 *CFR* 409.31.

96.   42 *USC* 1395(a)(1)(A).

97.   42 *CFR* 409.35.

[98]. 42 *CFR* 435.914; *Medi-Cal Eligibility Procedure Manual*, Letter #140; and *ACWDL* #95-17.

[99]. 42 *U.S.C.* 1396p, as adopted in *California Welfare & Institutions Code* §14009.5, and 22 *California Code of Regulations* §50960.

[100]. *Statement of Facts Supporting Medi-Cal Application of Patient in a Long Term Care Facility*, Question 17A.

[101]. *Probate Code* §215.

[102]. *Probate Code* §9202.

About the Author

F. Bentley Mooney, Jr. is a North Hollywood attorney engaged in a business and estates law practice. *Business* law includes entity formation, dissolution and recapitalization, as well as transactions and related taxation. *Estates* law includes estate planning, Medi-Cal eligibility planning, asset protection planning for high net worth individuals, trusts, probate administration and related taxation.

Mr. Mooney entered the private practice of law in 1972. He has a Master of Laws (Taxation), is listed by Martindale-Hubbell in its *Bar Registry of Preeminent Lawyers*, holds a skills and ethics rating of *a-v* from Martindale-Hubbell, and is a frequent speaker on topics within his areas of practice concentration.

Mr. Mooney is also the author of numerous articles and books. Among the latter are *Handcuff the Tax Man, Going Bare, The Artful Use of Offshore Tax Havens, Cluster! A Flexible Approach to the Cluster Agency Maze,*

When Health is Lost: Providing for Long-Term Nursing Care (updated in this -- his eighth -- book), *Creating & Preserving Wealth, Preserving Your Wealth* and *Critical Planning for Target Defendants*.

Mr. Mooney receives calls for expert comment from *Forbes*, *Medical Economics*, *The Los Angeles Business Journal*, *Wall Street Journal* and more than a dozen other publications.

Mr. Mooney writes and publishes two newsletters for clients and friends of the firm. *FBM Report* is published quarterly and deals with general business and estates law. *FBM on Creating & Preserving Wealth* is published semi-annually and addresses asset protection issues for high net worth individuals.

Professional associations in which Mr. Mooney has held leadership positions include the Los Angeles County, California and American Bar Associations, Lawyers' Club of Los Angeles County, the (California) Conference of Bar Delegates and the Glendale Estate Planning Council. He is also a member of the National Academy of Elder Law Attorneys.

Mr. Mooney may be contacted at:

4605 Lankershim Boulevard, Suite 718
North Hollywood, California 91602
Telephone (818) 769-4221
Facsimile (818) 769-5002
e-mail fbmooney@pacbell.net
Worldwide Web
http://www.bentlymooney.com

www.ingramcontent.com/pod-product-compliance
Lightning Source LLC
Chambersburg PA
CBHW030429290526
45786CB00001B/205